The Rules of Recovery - Surviving Severe Depression and Anxiety

Mark Davenport

Published by Mark Davenport, 2023.

THE RULES OF RECOVERY - SURVIVING SEVERE DEPRESSION AND ANXIETY

First edition. May 15, 2023.

Copyright © 2023 Mark Davenport.

ISBN: 979-8223376576

Written by Mark Davenport.

BEFORE WE BEGIN

Depression is a serious mental illness that can have a profound impact on a person's daily life, and unfortunately, it is not always easy to identify. Many people who suffer from severe depression often go undetected by those around them because they work hard to hide their symptoms and maintain a façade of normalcy.

It is common for people with depression to experience feelings of hopelessness, worthlessness, and intense sadness, which can be overwhelming and debilitating. These feelings may be accompanied by physical symptoms such as fatigue, difficulty sleeping or oversleeping, and changes in appetite. In some cases, depression can lead to suicidal thoughts or behaviors.

Despite the severity of these symptoms, people with depression often put on a brave face and try to hide their struggles from those around them. They may feel ashamed or embarrassed about their feelings, and worry that they will be judged or misunderstood if they talk about them. This can make it difficult for others to recognize that they are suffering.

It is also worth noting that not everyone experiences depression in the same way. While some people may seem visibly upset or withdrawn, others may appear to be functioning normally on the surface, even as they struggle with intense emotional pain.

For those who are struggling with suicidal thoughts, the decision to hide their feelings can be particularly dangerous. They may feel like they have no one to turn to or that their loved ones will not understand their pain. In some cases, they may even be actively planning their suicide, carefully considering the methods they could use and weighing the consequences of their actions.

While it is not always possible to know when someone is suffering from depression, there are some signs that can be cause for concern. If you notice that a loved one seems to be withdrawing from activities they used to enjoy, expressing feelings of hopelessness or worthlessness, or exhibiting changes in behavior, such as increased irritability or aggression, it may be worth checking in with them to see how they are doing.

It is important to remember that depression is a real illness, and it is not a sign of weakness or a personal failing. If you or someone you know is struggling with depression, there is help available. Encourage them to seek support from a mental health professional, or consider reaching out to a crisis hotline or other resources for support. With the right treatment and support, it is possible to manage depression and regain a sense of hope and happiness.

If you have recently entertained thoughts of self-harm or have been preoccupied with ideations of taking your own life, I implore you to take action now. Reach out to someone you trust, no matter how daunting it may seem, and let them know what you are going through. Do not allow fear or shame to prevent you from seeking help. The resources for suicide prevention are numerous and accessible, including several helplines listed below.

Your presence here is valued, and I urge you to remain with us. I hope to witness you complete this journey and emerge as a stronger and healthier individual. Reading this book indicates that you are taking steps towards bettering yourself, but it is crucial to act upon these efforts. Contact a healthcare professional, a family member, or a friend - anyone who can provide you with the support you need. It is imperative that you do not delay any further.

You are an exceptionally unique and valuable individual, with a purpose that extends far beyond your current struggles. You are a one-in-ten-trillion chance, and it is imperative that you recognize your worth. Perhaps your purpose is to become someone who, like me, helps and saves others. Do not deprive the world of your potential; seek help and allow someone else to take the wheel, guiding you to a better place.

"I am now more educated about those signs, but they were symptoms of a man who was fighting his demons, but I had no idea how serious it was," Talinda Bennington said on CNN. "We just thought he was being a rock star."

Despite hoping that someone will recognize the pain and intervene, it is unfortunately common for individuals to miss the subtle signs of someone struggling with mental illness. Even I, personally, was able to hide my own pain from those closest to me, including my wife and psychologist. It often takes reaching a breaking point before finally opening up, resulting in increased medical treatment and time off work.

Society tends to downplay mental illness, and people often hesitate to speak up about their struggles for fear of being a burden or bringing others down. Although people may acknowledge the importance of mental health awareness and empathy, they may still deny or dismiss what they see in loved ones who are struggling. It can be an uncomfortable road for someone to intervene, fearing that they may be rejected or damage their relationship. Ultimately, it is up to the individual in distress to lower their shields, become vulnerable, and seek help.

Seek help

I cannot stress this enough - if you are experiencing dark thoughts or are in trouble, it is time to put this book down and take action. Reach out to someone you trust, whether it be by making a call or having a conversation with a friend or partner in the same room. It can be challenging to start the conversation, so I have included below some suggested narratives to help you ask for help in a way that minimizes embarrassment and shock. The important thing is to take action and seek help now.

Approach 1: Script: "Hey, I wanted to talk to you about something serious that's been on my mind. Lately, I've been feeling really overwhelmed and I'm having thoughts of hurting myself. I know it's difficult to hear, but I wanted to open up to you and get some help."

Approach 2: Script: "I've been feeling really down lately and I think I need to talk to someone about it. I've been having some thoughts of ending my life and I don't want to keep it to myself anymore. Can we talk about it?"

Approach 3: Script: "I'm feeling really lost and struggling to cope with everything. I've been having thoughts of self-harm and it's starting to scare me. I know it's not an easy conversation, but I want to reach out and ask for your support."

Approach 4: Script: "I've been feeling really low lately and I think it's time I opened up about what's been going on. I've been having some dark thoughts and I'm scared about where they might lead me. Can we talk about it?"

Approach 5: Script: "I wanted to talk to you about something that's been weighing heavily on my mind. Lately, I've been struggling with my mental health and it's starting to affect my ability to cope. I'm having thoughts of hurting myself and I know I need to reach out and ask for help. Can you be there for me?"

These approaches aim to start the conversation in a gentle and non-threatening way, limiting shame, embarrassment, and shock. It's important to remember that opening up about mental health struggles can be challenging, but seeking help is a courageous step towards healing.

Absolutely, if you have friends or loved ones who are struggling with mental health issues, it can be challenging to know how to support them. There are many resources available to help guide you in how to best approach these conversations and support those who are struggling.

One excellent resource is the website of the National Suicide Prevention Lifeline, which provides guidance on how to support someone who may be at risk of suicide. They offer tips on how to recognize warning signs, how to approach the conversation, and how to connect someone with the resources they need.

Here is the link to the National Suicide Prevention Lifeline's page on best practices for dealing with someone who may be thinking of suicide or hurting themselves due to depression: https://suicidepreventionlifeline.org/how-we-can-all-prevent-suicide/#supporting-someone

I hope this helps and encourages individuals to seek help and support for themselves or their loved ones. Remember, reaching out for help is a courageous step towards healing.

There are many warning signs and risk factors for mental health issues, including depression and suicidal thoughts. Here are ten questions to consider that, if answered "yes" to any three, could indicate that an individual should seek immediate help:

1. Have you been feeling persistently sad, hopeless, or empty?

2. Have you lost interest in activities that you used to enjoy?

3. Have you experienced changes in appetite, weight, or sleep patterns?

4. Have you been feeling irritable, agitated, or restless?

5. Have you been feeling fatigued or lacking energy?

6. Have you been feeling worthless or excessively guilty?

7. Have you been having difficulty concentrating, making decisions, or remembering things?

8. Have you been having thoughts of death or suicide?

9. Have you been engaging in self-harm behaviors or have you attempted suicide in the past?

10. Have you been experiencing physical symptoms such as headaches, stomach aches, or body aches without an apparent physical cause?

If an individual answers "yes" to any three of these questions, it could indicate that they are at risk for depression, suicidal thoughts, or other mental health issues. Seeking immediate help from a medical professional or mental health provider is strongly advised in such cases. It is always better to err on the side of caution and seek help, rather than ignore the warning signs and risk a potentially dangerous situation.

It is true that mental health has become a popular topic of discussion in recent years, with more and more people expressing their willingness to help those who are struggling. However, it is also true that some individuals may only be paying lip service to these issues, without truly understanding or addressing the underlying problems.

In some cases, individuals may be more interested in projecting a certain image of themselves as caring and compassionate, rather than actually taking meaningful action to help those in need. This can be particularly frustrating for those who are struggling with mental illness, as it may lead to missed opportunities for support and intervention.

It is important to remember that mental illness can affect anyone, regardless of age, gender, or socioeconomic status. It is not something that can be neatly compartmentalized or ignored simply because it is uncomfortable or inconvenient. While it is easy to make promises or express virtuous sentiments, it is much harder to follow through with real, substantive action.

That being said, there are also many individuals who genuinely care about mental health and are willing to do whatever they can to help those in need. These individuals may not be the most vocal or public about their efforts, but their actions speak louder than words. It is important to recognize and appreciate these individuals for their genuine compassion and willingness to help.

In the end, mental health is a complex and multifaceted issue that requires ongoing attention and support. It is important to remain vigilant and mindful of the ways in which we can all contribute to creating a more supportive and compassionate environment for those who are struggling.

If you are still reading this, it is likely that you are searching for help and support for your mental health struggles. It takes courage to acknowledge that you need help and to take steps towards getting it. Trust me, you are not alone, and there are resources available to you that can help you overcome your challenges and find a path towards healing.

One of the most important things you can do for yourself right now is to form a support team. This may include family members, friends, a therapist, a support group, or other mental health professionals. These individuals can provide you with emotional support, guidance, and resources to help you manage your mental health and work towards recovery. Remember, it is okay to ask for help and to lean on others when you need it.

It is also important to take care of your physical health during this time. If you are drinking or using drugs that have not been prescribed for you, it is time to stop. Substance use can worsen mental health symptoms and make it harder to manage your mental health challenges. Instead, focus on engaging in healthy behaviors such as exercise, getting enough sleep, and eating a balanced diet.

Remember, seeking help for mental health struggles is a sign of strength, not weakness. You deserve to feel happy, healthy, and fulfilled, and with the right support and resources, you can achieve these goals. Take the first step towards healing today and reach out for help.*f*

Of course, here's a brief summary of the key findings and concepts from each of the mentioned papers:

1. Frodl & O'Keane (2013): This review paper discusses the effects of cumulative stress on the brain, with a particular focus on developmental stress, HPA axis function, and hippocampal structure. The authors highlight that prolonged stress and severe depression can lead to alterations in the hypothalamic-pituitary-adrenal (HPA) axis, which regulates the stress response. These alterations can cause changes in the hippocampus, a brain region involved in learning and memory. The paper suggests that early-life stress may have long-lasting effects on brain structure and function, increasing the risk of developing depression and other psychiatric disorders.

2. MacQueen & Frodl (2011): This paper reviews the evidence for the role of the hippocampus in major depression, discussing the convergence of preclinical and clinical research. The authors report that individuals with major depression often exhibit smaller hippocampal volumes, which may be related to the duration and severity of depression. They also highlight the importance of early intervention and treatment, as it may help prevent or reverse these structural changes in the brain.

3. Sheline et al. (1999): In this study, the authors investigated the relationship between depression duration, age, and hippocampal volume in medically healthy women with recurrent major depression. The results showed that longer depression duration was associated with greater hippocampal volume loss, but age did not have a significant effect. This finding emphasizes the importance of timely treatment for depression to potentially prevent long-lasting changes in brain structure.

4. Treadway & Zald (2011): This review paper focuses on anhedonia, the loss of pleasure or interest in previously enjoyable activities, which is a core symptom of major depression. The authors discuss the relevance of translational neuroscience for understanding the neurobiological basis of anhedonia and its relationship to depression. They argue that a better understanding of the neural circuits and mechanisms underlying anhedonia may help identify new treatment targets for depression and improve our understanding of the long-term consequences of the disorder.

In summary, these papers highlight the potential long-lasting effects of severe depression on the brain, particularly in relation to hippocampal structure, HPA axis function, and anhedonia. They emphasize the importance of early intervention and treatment to potentially prevent or reverse these changes and improve long-term outcomes.

The long-lasting effects of severe depression on the brain can manifest in various ways in an individual, including changes in cognitive function, emotional regulation, and stress response. Here, I'll expand on these potential consequences as they relate to heightened focus on learning and memory issues.

1. Hippocampal structure: As mentioned in the papers, prolonged stress and depression can lead to changes in the hippocampus, a brain region involved in learning and memory. Smaller hippocampal volume has been associated with depression, and this change may be more pronounced in individuals with longer durations of depression or more severe symptoms. This reduction in hippocampal volume can result in memory impairments, such as difficulty in consolidating new memories, retrieving old memories, or spatial navigation. However, it is important to note that not all individuals with depression will experience these memory issues, and the severity can vary.

2. HPA axis function: Prolonged stress and depression can also cause alterations in the hypothalamic-pituitary-adrenal (HPA) axis, which regulates the stress response. This dysregulation can lead to heightened cortisol levels, which can have detrimental effects on the brain, including the hippocampus. High cortisol levels have been associated with cognitive impairments, such as difficulties in attention, concentration, and learning. However, once again, the impact on cognitive function can vary between individuals and may not necessarily result in a heightened focus on learning.

3. Anhedonia and motivation: Anhedonia, the loss of pleasure or interest in previously enjoyable activities, is a core symptom of major depression. This can lead to reduced motivation, which in turn can affect learning and memory. A lack of motivation might make it difficult for individuals with depression to engage in learning activities, concentrate on tasks, or put forth the effort required to encode and retrieve memories effectively. As a result, learning and memory might suffer due to decreased engagement and motivation.

While the long-lasting effects of depression on the brain can result in memory impairments and difficulties in attention and concentration, it is essential to keep in mind that these consequences can vary between individuals. Some people might experience more subtle or mild cognitive changes, while others might have more pronounced deficits. It's also important to note that early intervention and treatment for depression can help mitigate these effects and improve long-term outcomes.

It is important to note that I am an AI language model and not a mental health professional. I can provide some general insights based on the information given, but for personalized advice or recommendations, please consult a healthcare professional.

In the case of an individual who has experienced two severe episodes of depression involving self-harm, and who is now medicated with Trintellix, Rexulti, and Vyvanse, several factors could impact their personality, learning, and hyperfocus:

1. Medication effects: The medications mentioned (Trintellix, Rexulti, and Vyvanse) can have different effects on the individual's mood, cognition, and behavior. Trintellix is an antidepressant that may improve mood, energy levels, and feelings of well-being. Rexulti is an atypical antipsychotic that is sometimes used as an adjunct treatment for major depressive disorder, and it can help improve mood and reduce anxiety. Vyvanse is a stimulant medication primarily prescribed for ADHD, which may help improve attention, focus, and executive function. The combined effect of these medications may result in improvements in mood and cognitive function, potentially leading to positive changes in personality, learning, and attention.

2. ADHD and executive function: The presence of ADHD can impact an individual's attention, impulsivity, and executive function, which in turn can affect their personality, learning, and focus. It is important to consider the potential interactions between ADHD and depression, as both conditions can have overlapping cognitive and emotional symptoms. A highly developed executive function, however, may help mitigate some of the challenges associated with ADHD, allowing the individual to better manage their symptoms and develop effective coping strategies.

3. Recovery and resilience: The experience of severe depression and self-harm can have lasting effects on an individual's mental health, cognition, and overall well-being. As the individual recovers from these episodes, they may experience changes in their personality, learning abilities, and focus. Factors such as effective treatment, support networks, and personal resilience can play a crucial role in recovery and long-term outcomes.

4. Personal variability: It's essential to recognize that the effects of depression, ADHD, and medications can vary significantly between individuals. Some people may experience more pronounced changes in their personality, learning, and focus, while others may have more subtle or even positive changes.

In summary, the individual's personality, learning abilities, and focus could be impacted by several factors, including the effects of medication, the presence of ADHD, the recovery process from depressive episodes, and personal variability. It is crucial to work closely with a healthcare professional to monitor progress, adjust medications as needed, and develop personalized strategies to manage mental health and cognitive function.

FORWARD & DEDICATION

Welcome to my story - one that I had never imagined myself writing, especially during the darkest moments of my mental health crisis. Through this book, I hope to provide an easy-to-understand and concise account of my struggles and my journey to overcoming them. I'm not cured yet, but I'm doing much better, and I want to be a beacon of hope to others who may be dealing with similar circumstances. I don't think we are ever "cured", like an alcoholic, we must remain vigilant and watchful for those signs of trouble. The culmination of this book is dedicated to my wife Eve, who was my rock. Without her understanding, love, and undying support, I'm not sure I would have been able to make it through. I'm also very thankful for my family and friends, even my work buddy (you know who you are) for helping me along the way.

So why should someone consider reading a self-help book? It's no secret that professional help can be expensive, especially if there is an extended period of treatment required. But then, what is expensive when some people can spend thousands of dollars a year on alcohol or, worse, cigarettes that harm the body but will resist and or complain about spending money on something that will truly help them and possibly save their lives? Self-help books offer an affordable, convenient and accessible alternative to introducing oneself to self-care and managing mental health condition. Authors of these books are often experts in the field, or have gone through what they are writing about. They can provide readers with portable, valuable information and insight into their mental health and step-by-step techniques on how to manage it. Someone in therapy could greatly benefit from the self-reflection such books can provide and the resulting in empowering of people to take a more active role in their recovery. To illustrate this point further, renowned psychologist like Jordan Peterson, Aaron T. Beck, Marsha Linehan and Robert Sapolsky highlight the positive effects of self-help books and how it can supplement professional treatments. It's almost like going on a quest together, where the reader and I bring in pieces of the same puzzle. We are teaming up against our demons, learning to understand and conquer them, one step at a time.

THE STATISTICS ON DEPRESSION

Depression is a serious and increasingly common mental health concern that affects people of all ages and genders. Statistics from the World Health Organization (WHO) state that depression is the world's leading cause of disability, affecting millions annually. Across different populations, the prevalence of depression can vary - with women generally being at greater risk than men, while those aged 60 and over having the highest risk overall. Unfortunately, many children and adolescents also struggle with depression at rates of 3-5% and 8-12% respectively. It is important to recognize that people may exhibit different symptoms of depression that may not always be recorded in official statistics. Anyone at any age can develop depression, and it is important to seek help if you find that you are experiencing symptoms.

Even with knowledge of the prevalence of depression, it can still be a daunting and complex mental health issue to tackle. Thankfully, there are a plethora (I love that word, plethora) of self-help books available to assist people with managing their mental health. However, not all mental health books are particularly helpful, so it is important to know which characteristics to look for in an effective book. A good self-help book should be evidence-based, include practical strategies, be written using language that is accessible to the reader and be tailored to their individual needs and circumstances. Fortunately, renowned psychologists such as Aaron T. Beck, Jordan Peterson, Robert Sapolsky and Marsha Linehan have written self-help books that meet these criteria and can help individuals approach depression more effectively.

It can be helpful to think of reading self-help mental health books as akin to putting together a jigsaw puzzle. Reading different books – like searching for the pieces of the puzzle – can give us a sense of our mental health issue, create useful insights and form new perspectives. Only when all the pieces come together, can the complete picture of depression can be seen and can a pathway to successful management of mental health be formulated.

WHAT MAKES A GOOD SELF-HELP BOOK

A comprehensive self-help book on mental health should be a guide for its readers, empowering them to take control of their recovery. An effective book should provide accurate, reliable information that is easy to understand and free of unnecessary jargon while giving practical, actionable advice and techniques on managing mental health issues. Before choosing a self-help book on mental health, it is advisable to read through the reviews and find one written by experienced mental health professionals, such as psychologists or psychiatrists, who can recommend it as a dependable source or a knowledgeable author who has experienced the disease, someone who has indeed been through the journey and followed the advice they provide. In the case of this book, I fall in the later, as I am not a doctor but have experienced severe depression and anxiety and have sought professional help. I have also spend hundreds of hours on research, reading hundreds of peer-reviewed studies on various topics relating to depression and anxiety, so although not formally educated, I have become quite proficient in cognitive behaviour therapy and many of the methods used to treat depression and anxiety.

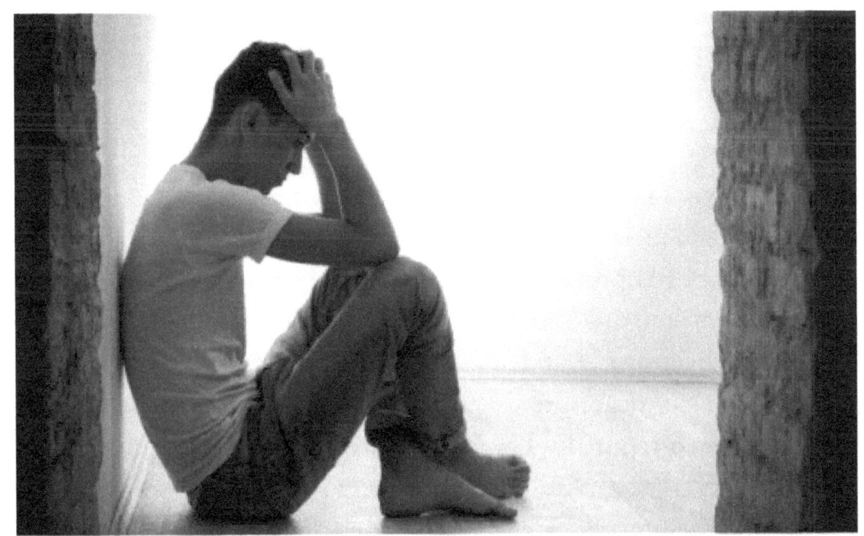

A good self-help book should not offer a 'quick-fix', but instead offer a balanced approach to dealing with mental health concerns. It should also encourage readers to accept responsibility for their own improvement, providing them with a sense of empowerment and understanding. For example, Jordan Peterson's 12 Rules for Life: An Antidote to Chaos is a great example of a self-help book on mental health, as it explains the science behind anxiety and depression and provides readers with practical resources and advice on how to manage and control their mental health.

At the same time, it is essential to recognize when a mental health condition needs more than self-help. For instance, in cases of severe depression or anxiety, it is recommended to see a psychologist or psychiatrist. Therapy and medications, when clinically recommended, can help to reduce symptoms, but ultimately, the individual must still take an active role in maintaining and improving mental health. As Robert Sapolsky puts it, "The self is not an isolated entity..it is collaborative, effortful and perpetual." A self-help book on mental health can be seen as a tool to help facilitate collaboration, effort and perseverance.

ESSENTIAL CONSIDERATIONS TO RECOVERY

Therapy: Talking to a therapist or counselor can help individuals understand their depression and develop strategies for coping with it. My experience has proven this to be true. If you are suffering from severe depression and or anxiety, I would suggest a psychologist.

Medication: Antidepressant medication can help to alleviate symptoms of depression, such as feelings of sadness, hopelessness, and lack of energy. Initially, I tried to avoid prescriptions, but once things did not progress as we had hoped, I involved a psychiatrist who prescribed me the medications I needed. Your psychologist will be able to best advise you.

Exercise: Engaging in regular exercise is a great way to boost your mood and reduce symptoms of depression. Whether it's going for a long walk, doing yoga, or finding activities that fit into how you're feeling, anything is better than nothing. Plus, physical activity can help increase the production of endorphins, which are natural mood elevators that can help reduce feelings of depression, anxiety, and stress.

When engaging in physical activity and witnessing improvements in physical fitness, people may experience a heightened sense of self-esteem and worth. Achieving even small fitness goals can bring a sense of accomplishment and satisfaction, which can be beneficial for mental health. Additionally, regular exercise can help to improve the quality of sleep, which is essential for overall health and can help with depression and anxiety symptoms. Finally, physical activity can reduce physical symptoms of stress, such as tension headaches, muscle aches, and fatigue.

Physical activity can be a great way to distract from negative thoughts and feelings, which can be beneficial for managing mental health issues. It can also help to regulate emotions and lessen symptoms of anxiety and depression. It's important to remember that physical activity should be part of a larger treatment plan, and it's important to work with a mental health professional to determine the best type and frequency of exercise that is right for you.

Adequate Sleep: To ensure optimal health and wellbeing, it is essential to get enough restful sleep. Social Support: Having a supportive network of family and friends can be a great aid in managing depression, as they can provide emotional support and motivation. This for me having ADHD is always a struggle in that my mind, once it stirs in the morning I usually cannot go back to sleep.

Self-Care: Engaging in activities that bring joy and relaxation, such as yoga, meditation, journaling and reading, can be beneficial in managing depression. It is important to note that everyone's recovery from depression is different, and it is important to work with a mental health professional to create a personalized treatment plan.

Negative thoughts and self-talk: Do you find yourself feeling bad about yourself or putting yourself down? Do you struggle with negative thoughts and self-talk, remaining in a state of high negativity? These are all symptoms of depression, leading to low self-esteem and a lack of enthusiasm for life.

Low Energy: You may find yourself wanting to stay in bed all day, struggling to find motivation to do even the simplest of tasks. You may even find yourself getting upset easily, and feeling like the world is a terrible place. In addition, you may find yourself taking potentially harmful risks to yourself or others, as your feelings of hopelessness and despair can cause you to act out. This can lead to hurting the people you love most and reacting with frustration and anger to simple things. If you experience any of these symptoms, it is important to reach out for help.

Isolation: You may not feel like venturing out or being around people, even virtually. You might feel lonely, yet at the same time not want to be around people. It's like you yearn for company but you don't want to be too close. This could lead to you isolating yourself by avoiding spending time with family and friends. This was a real struggle for me because I felt that being with family would make me feel better, but it was so hard to get there. This caused a lot of tension between my wife and I as she was understanding, but depression is so hard to comprehend for those around you. I often wished they could spend a day in my head and quickly understand the agony.

Dwelling on the bad: You may think about all the bad things in life or painful memories from the past. When you are not in a positive state of mind it is easy to focus on the negative. You may ruminate over bad situations to the point where you are mentally exhausted. This only adds to the need to isolate more. Depression is incredibly complex, making it a tough illness to deal with.

Living an unhealthy lifestyle: You may choose to skip meals, eat junk food, stop exercising, or stop wearing a mask as you no longer care about your health. This is easy to do when you need more energy to get groceries and you are relying on fast food. It is important to remember that your health can have an effect on your anxiety and depression, so it is important to take care of your body by eating healthy.

Exercise

Exercising regularly can help promote positive mental health in numerous ways. It releases endorphins which can increase cheerful and relaxed feelings, while also improving an individual's physical fitness. Working towards fitness goals can be particularly beneficial, as they can bring a sense of accomplishment and satisfaction which can be good for mood. Furthermore, studies done by psychologists like Jordan Peterson, Aaron T. Beck, Marsha Linehan, and Robert Sapolsky, have found that regular physical activity can decrease feelings of depression, anxiety, and stress. It can also improve the quality of sleep, which is important for overall wellbeing, regulating negative emotions and reducing physical stress symptoms such as fatigue, muscle aches and tension headaches.

Finally, engaging in physical activities can be distracting for those with depression and anxiety, providing a momentary reprieve from negative thoughts and feelings. This can be beneficial when part of a larger treatment plan. However, it is not a replacement as proper mental health therapy is also essential. Additionally, it is important to pay attention to other elements of mental health, like getting adequate restful sleep, surrounding oneself with supportive networks, and engaging in self-care activities to bring joy and relaxation. Negative thoughts and self-talk can also be obvious symptoms of depression, which can lead to low self-esteem and a lack of ambition. To better manage depression and its symptoms, it is best to have a personalized treatment plan crafted with the help of a mental health professional.

To illustrate, when dealing with mental health, things like exercising, positive self-talk, and healthy lifestyle decisions can be likened to building a house. We cannot just build a roof and a door, if we don't have a foundation. Therefore, the foundation is drawn from a mental health professional's expertise, upon which the rest can be built. Exercising, engaging in self-care activities, building networks of support, and regular sleep can be the further building blocks, helping to build a strong sense of overall mental health.

Low energy

Depression and isolation can be a devastating combination. Feeling drained and lacking in motivation, being on edge and easily upset, and acting out in potentially dangerous ways can all be signs of depression that need attention. Additionally, those who suffer from depression often find themselves wanting company yet not wanting to reach out, preferring to isolate themselves from family, friends and loved ones. Such disconnection can flow from a tendency to focus on the negative, ruminating on bad experiences, which further sucks energy, making it difficult to even make the effort to get out of bed. Finally, those suffering from depression may develop unhealthy habits when it comes to food, exercise, or refraining from taking important measures to take care of themselves, such as mask-wearing.

It can be incredibly difficult for those around us to comprehend how such a dark feeling can consume a person. This is a thought echoed by numerous leading psychologists; for example, Jordan Peterson talks about depression being like a 'black cloud', whereas Aaron T. Beck discusses the cognitive distortions that come with being depressed. Marsha Linehan equates it to burning a candle from both ends, taking from little resources to reach a task and then expecting the same level of performance. Similarly, Robert Sapolsky explains how the physiology of depression changes how we view the world, making it difficult to make well-informed decisions.

The message is clear; depression is a serious mental health issue that can harm our lifestyle habits. It's important to remember that depression is an illness, not a flaw and that professional help is available. We can liken it to a battery running low. If we don't prioritize recharging, it can cause long-term damage that is hard to repair. Taking steps to better our mental health and seek appropriate help can help us get to a point where we can lead more fulfilling and healthy life.

TRIGGER WARNING

WARNING – READER DISCRETION IS ADVISED. THIS CHAPTER COULD BE TRIGGERING FOR SOME. IF YOU ARE NOT IN A GOOD PLACE AT THIS TIME, IT IS RECOMMENDED TO SKIP THIS CHAPTER. IT IS ONLY INCLUDED AS BACKGROUND INFORMATION AND IS NOT NEEDED TO GAIN THE BENEFITS OF THIS BOOK. DARK DAYS – WHEN IT ALL WENT WRONG

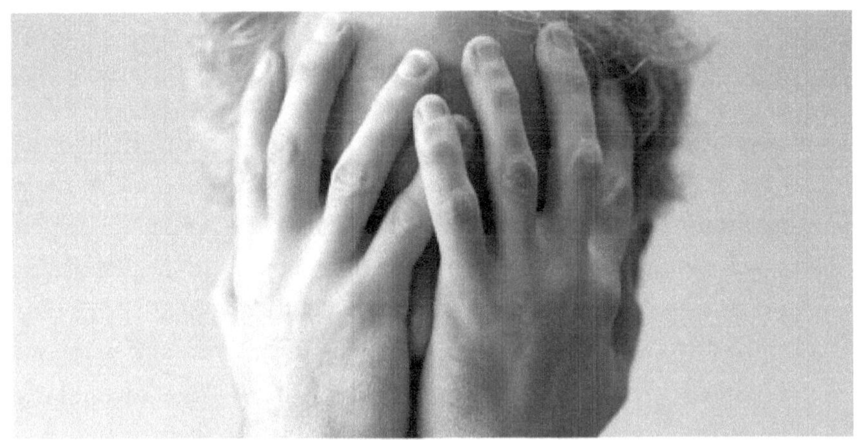

The Dark Days

It was 2017 and it seem the years of battling whatever life had thrown at me along the last several decades had finally fatigued me to the point that I was nearly broken beyond repair. I was never a one to reach out for help due to the stigma often attached to mental health challenges, and so I pushed back down my struggles and silently grappled with every day. I started to distance myself from family and friends and subsequently felt alone in whatever storm I was dwelling in. For years I would take on more battle scars and would almost say to life, "is that the best you can do?" I felt no matter how bad things got, and they got pretty bloody bad at times, I would go into this auto-pilot mode and somehow dig myself out. But this time, it was different in that after months of failing to cope with the magnitude of my issues, after much prodding from my wife, I finally chose to seek outside assistance. Often, these types of decisions are met with hesitation, but this was now different, this was me literally fighting for my life, and I knew that I had to act before it deteriorated to a very unhappy ending. Desperately, I sought out my employer's Employee Assistance Program, and soon as I worked with them, as good as they were, it became apparent to both them and myself that I needed more specialized help, and I needed it soon.

I was introduced to several psychologists, psychiatrists, and my family doctor through connections. It was a very beneficial decision, and I was soon seeing a specialist multiple times a month and even occasionally daily. With pretty well known expers in the field who spoke about depression like Jordan Peterson to Aaron T. Beck, Marsha Linehan and Robert Sapolsky who impacted me the most at the time, each of them imparted various doses of wisdom, assurance, and tremendous amounts of insight into what I was experiencing. In short, they had become my virtual family; the lighthouse of hope that help fuel the pillars of my recovery. Much like a boat at sea, when one encounters choppy waters and all the riches of the deep, sometimes it takes a crew of professionals to get the vessel safely back to shore.

The concept of seeking help for mental health may still feel overwhelming and uncertain for some, so it is important to note that this is a perfectly normal feeling for any journey of self-discovery. Human development is a slow and winding road, and not everyone needs the same assistance to get where they're headed. Find the people and resources that are suited to your specific needs and tap into their knowledge, as they may just be your saving grace.

Being diagnosed with anxiety and depression was a turning point in my life; it was an overwhelming state of feeling lost and helplessness. I had been struggling with this without knowing what it was or how bad it was about to be. Every day felt like a battle that I could never win, and I was terrified of where it would end up taking me. I would often not eat, stay in all day, and isolate myself from loved ones, making me feel terrible for doing so. All of this was compounded by the negative self-talk and guilt that comes along with depression.

My anxiety consisted of worrying about the worst-case outcomes of various situations, heart palpitations, an upset stomach, and middle-of-the-night panic attacks. These were extremely frightening events that left me feeling unable to breathe and often accompanied by a cold sweat and soaked clothing. Thankfully, I was able to get help from a new clinician, my own personal Psychologist, who I will call Dr. P who to this day help me manage my anxiety and depression more effectively. I swear she knows me better than I know myself. She was not only a phycologist, she was incredibly intelligent and had this innate ability to pick up on the most subtle ques as well, I could not snow her, as she was far well too armed in her skills for that to happen. For me, I hit the jackpot since I know now, she is so busy, it would be all but impossible to seek her out to be my psychologist. Before we go further, I will do my best to frame things up a bit in terms of depression and anxiety, not so much from a clinical view, but more from a view of someone who lived it.

It is extremely important to me that when someone is reading this and I give suggestions, they don't think, "Oh easy for you to say." Things always look better on paper than the sometimes do in practice, but the things I suggest, I realize some may work for you and some may not, but the overarching message is indeed your compass to safety.

It's important to consider that anxiety and depression are like enemy forces trying to control our well-being and happiness. They can drive us to such a dark place if we let them. It's essential that we recognize and address these issues healthily and safely. For example, if a big problem arises, we should approach it analytically rather than catastrophizing or allowing it to consume our thoughts. It's like having your car break down, and instead of reaching the conclusion that your engine will never work again, you try to fix the problem step by step. This mindset helps us identify the problem, come up with solutions, and solve them one at a time. This helps to break the cycle of anxiety and depression instead of letting it become a vortex of negative feelings.

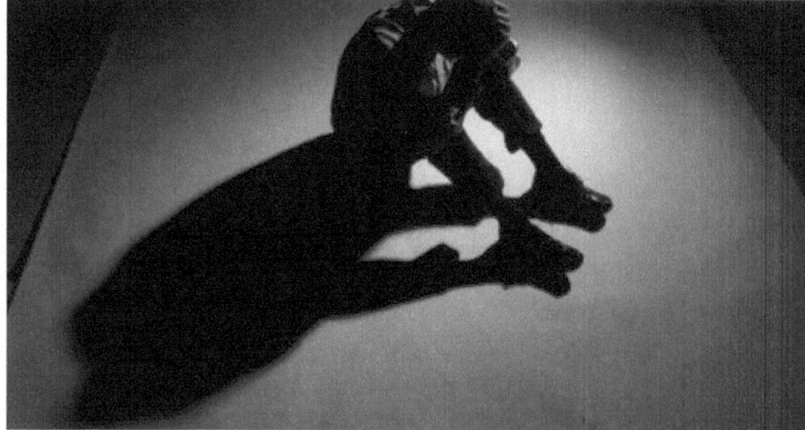

As I lived through my depression, I gradually felt more withdrawn, insecure, and helpless – my emotional and psychological condition was deteriorating. At three distinct moments, my depression had become so severe that I was pushed to the brink of despair. I had no choice but to make painful and difficult confessions to those I loved, confessing my inner battles and insecurities. The guilt and shame which followed were unbearable, no matter how much empathy and compassion were offered. Additionally, my depression had caused me to form certain rules and beliefs which, unsurprisingly, weren't factual or accurate; I had to continuously remind myself not to act based on these false beliefs and thoughts. My daily life became an exhausting battle, as I was constantly trying to identify my cognitive distortions and change my mental perceptions of situations. It was like having to remember to keep breathing – a single wrong move could have resulted in catastrophic consequences, and it almost did.

Depression is an invisible ailment often not understood, leaving many to doubt its validity and impact. Its effects were not only impacting me, those close to me were also witness to my breakdowns, compounding the distress. In response to this state of affairs, I began writing 'Medicated'; a book intended to help facilitate understanding and provide insight into me and my mental condition. In my desperate attempt to get better, I began three psychiatric medications: Trintellix, Vyvanse, and Rexulti - each with their side effects and drawbacks. Though the process was not easy, I am now in a much better place and doing everything I can to ensure that my mental health remains resilient.

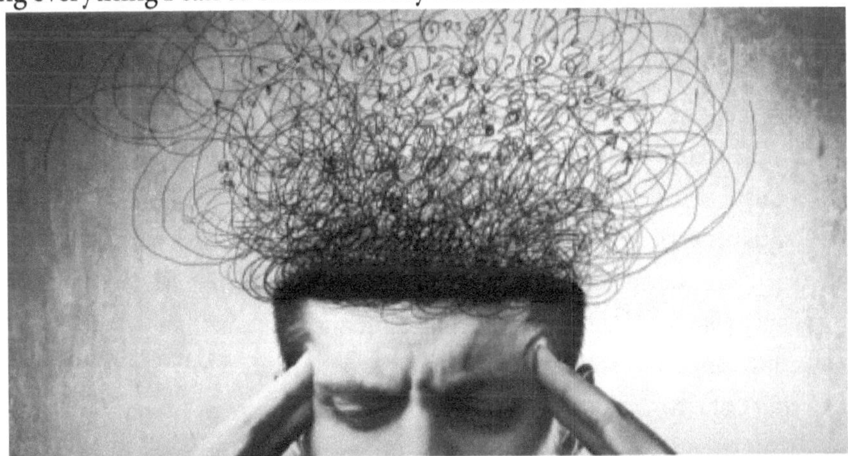

Depression is a multifaceted and multifarious illness, with symptoms differing between individuals and affected by myriad factors. It is not uncommon for depression patients to simultaneously deal with anxiety – a mental health disorder characterized by excessive worry, fear and trepidation towards uncertain or potential future occurrences and events. Depression is not just feeling sad; it is an invisible burden that can twist one's perception and transform the world around them into a hostile, unfamiliar place. Psychologists such Jordan Peterson, Aaron T. Beck, Marsha Linehan and Robert Sapolsky, have done considerable work on treating depression, using their knowledge and expertise to develop effective and successful therapy techniques. Mental illness can be likened to a stone - each having an invisible load that we carry with us through life, yet through proper care and patience, we can eventually learn to approach and move that stone.

The relationship between depression and anxiety is extremely complex, and it is important to understand the dynamic between the two for those dealing with either disorder. Research has revealed a bidirectional relationship between depression and anxiety, with one often being a progenitor of the other. According to the National Alliance on Mental Illness, individuals suffering from anxiety are three to five times more likely to experience depression than those without an anxiety disorder. Simultaneously, the World Health Organization states that those with depression commonly have symptoms of anxiety, such as feelings of fear, worry, and helplessness. Ultimately, this indicates a challenging cycle of reactions between depression and anxiety, with symptoms of both mental illnesses interweaving to form a unique and difficult experience.

For example, the constant fear and worry associated with anxiety can make it difficult to experience pleasure or any sign of joy. This may contribute to feelings of hopelessness, despair, and low mood – all classic traits of depression. In the reverse, the low mood and lack of motivation associated with depression can lead to physical symptoms such as fatigue, unintended changes in appetite and sleep, inferring a heightened degree of worry. And worry can very quickly lead to an anxiety disorder. It is clear then, that depression and anxiety are intrinsically linked, forming a complex relationship.

When it comes to treatment, renowned psychiatrist Jordan Peterson, among other top psychologists like Aaron T. Beck, Marsha Linehan, and Robert Sapolsky, advocates for a balanced approach that involves an even combination of medical support and cognitive-behavioural therapy. To make this approach even more effective, patients may often need to address issues of belief and meaning in life, which can be tricky with the help of a mental health professional. Indeed, this is where the patient can actively work on deconstructing the link between depression and anxiety and creating a healthier dialogue between the two. This is the journey I took where I dealt with a few of what they call your "core beliefs" that in my case were distorted, leading to many of the issues I faced. This was a long battle I worked with Dr. P on, where she and her expertise and knowledge as a psychologist got me through this incredibly difficult time. There were sessions where she would ask a question that would hit me like a lighting bolt as a feeling that was pushed down so deep for decades resurfaced like a bloated dead body, shocked and stirred incredibly powerful emotions. There was one such time when, in a session that my wife had joined me, Dr. P asked me about something in a way I had never been asked before, my emotional response was so powerful, I felt I was going to actually pass out. She had to offer me this mental stimulation technique to bring me down, it was simply incredible and scary as well all at the same time. This happened numerous times as we unraveled the decades of dysfunction, but once all the pieces were apart, we then started to correctly piece them and me back together, with newly formed core beliefs that would now govern my automatic thoughts.

In many ways, depression and anxiety can be likened to an uncomfortable game of tug of war, with each side seemingly inaccessible. To achieve a resolution, then, it is essential to have a comprehensive plan alongside an open dialogue to combat both illnesses more effectively.

Doing so can provide a safe space to acknowledge and process positive and negative emotions and offers a sense of reprieve from overwhelming mental battles.

Mental health issues such as depression and anxiety can be complicated and can easily spiral into a vicious cycle that can soon become unmanageable. It is essential for those experiencing these challenging conditions to seek help from a trained mental health professional in order to receive the appropriate treatment. Severe depression is an especially serious mental illness that affects millions of individuals globally and is characterized by persistent feelings of sadness, despair, and a complete loss of enjoyment from activities that once brought pleasure. Although it is imperative for people with depression to access professional help, many suffer in silence due to the shame and misunderstanding associated with mental health issues, making people hesitant to seek assistance or publicly know their struggles.

Hiding the symptoms of severe depression has serious and long-term implications. People may feel that they should be able to cope with their condition on their own, believing that asking for help is an indication of weakness, so they may try to put a brave face on things and act as if nothing is wrong. Yet, this tactic can easily lead to misunderstandings and strained relationships, and in some cases, even result in the breakdown of relationships if not managed properly. Furthermore, suppose people are not open about their struggles. In that case, they may not get the support and counselling they need to manage their symptoms and improve their quality of life, which can worsen their condition over time and in some cases result in deeply tragic consequences such as suicide.

People can hide the symptoms of their severe depression for various reasons. There is still a large amount of stigma surrounding mental health issues; some may be embarrassed or feel ashamed of their depression. They may worry that others will judge them or see them as weak if they open up about their struggles, particularly friends and family. Many may not even realize their symptoms are linked to depression, or not know how to articulate their feelings or ask for help. This is where mental health professionals, such as Jordan Peterson, Aaron T. Beck, Marsha Linehan and Robert Sapolsky, are essential. They are trained to help people understand, manage, and cope with the intricacies of severe depression, and provide the support and guidance individuals need to safely make the steps to getting better. In much the same way that a plumber has the skills to patch a leaky pipe, mental health professionals have the knowledge and experience to repair the troubled mind.

People may be hesitant to seek help for their depression due to fear of the consequences such as job loss, social isolation, or relationship problems, as well as not knowing where to turn for help or having access to mental health services. Furthermore, societal expectations have created a stigma that forces people to think they have to handle their issues independently, out of fear of seeming 'weak'. The World Health Organization (WHO) estimates that 4.4% of the global population, or 264 million people, suffer from depression, and it is projected to be the second leading cause of disability worldwide by 2020. While these numbers may differ country to country and population to population, it is important to remember that depression is a medical condition that can be treated, and seeking assistance is the first step to recovery. It is alright not to feel alright.

In order to help those who may be struggling with depression, here are 10 common symptoms to look out for: a loss of interest in activities that were once enjoyed, like sports, music, work, or social life; a lack of motivation; changes in sleep patterns; changes in appetite (which can be manifested as an increase or decrease, leading to potentially weight loss or gain); difficulty concentrating; feelings of guilt, worthlessness, and despair; loss of energy; thoughts of suicide or self-harm; and social withdrawal.

1. Loss of interest in activities that they once enjoyed, such as

sports, music, work, or social life.

2. Loss of enthusiasm for things they used to love.
3. Lack of motivation.
4. Changes in sleep patterns.
5. Changes in appetite.
6. Difficulty concentrating.
7. Feelings of worthlessness and guilt.
8. Loss of energy.
9. Thoughts of suicide or self-harm.
10. Social withdrawal.

Struggles With Abandonment:

Dr. Marsha Linehan, creator of Dialectical Behavior Therapy (DBT), has found that abandoning feelings are often strong components of depression. Those with depression feel like they are abandoned and alone, overwhelmed by despair and unable to find anyone who can relate to their feelings. They may feel like everyone else is living a happy life, while they are left to their own individual melancholia. An analogy that can illustrate this concept is that of a lighthouse. The lighthouse is alone at sea, the beacon of light can be seen for miles around but often those who are in its gaze are too far away to recognize or help an aid the pain it is harbouring deep within.

It is essential to remember that depression is a very real and serious issue, and seeking help is the best thing someone can do if they are dealing with symptoms of depression. Acknowledging and understanding the mental illness helps one and others worldwide who may be struggling to find hope in their darkest hour. Treatments of depression include many different kinds of therapies and medications, depending on the person and their condition. Jordan Peterson and Aaron T. Beck have advocated for cognitive behavior therapy while Robert Sapolsky has advocated for the usage of pharmaceuticals in combination with psychotherapy. Ultimately, anyone who is struggling with depression should seek help from mental healthcare professionals who can help guide them towards a successful recovery.

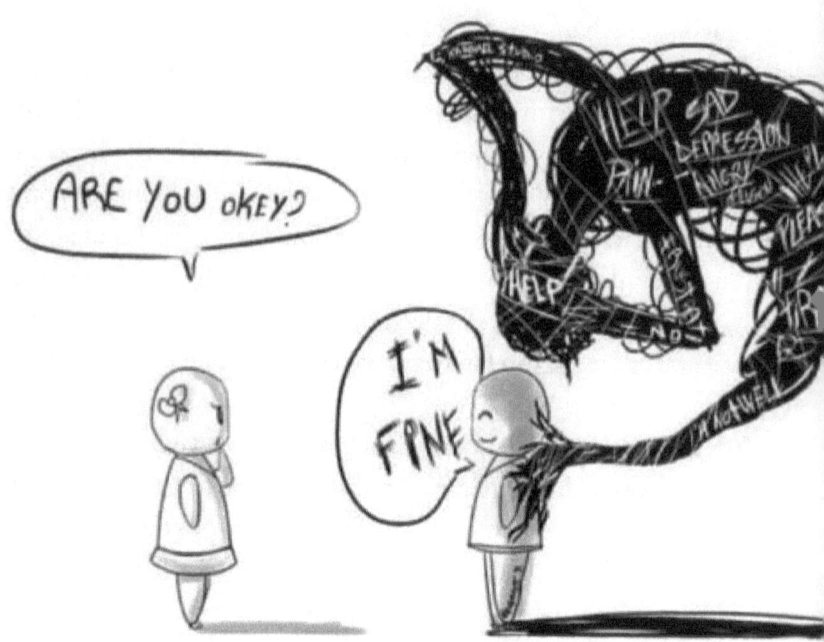
ARE YOU okEy?
I'M FINE
HELP
SAD
DEPRESSION
PAIN
ANGRY
HELP
PLE
NO

Abnormal Sleeping Habits:

Abnormal sleeping habits, such as insomnia and oversleeping, are tell-tale signs of depression. Those with depression can become adept at lying to maintain the 'I'm fine' facade and often distance themselves from others, choosing to spend most of their time alone. This perceived isolation can lead to a lack of motivation and a feeling of having no purpose. Furthermore, those with depression often begin to search for ways to alter their mental state through the use of either stimulating or depressant substances such as caffeine, sugar, alcohol or drugs.

The importance of recognizing signs of depression in individuals should not be underestimated. Jordan Peterson, the renowned psychologist and author, describes it as an 'enormous vulnerability; it's an invisible struggle, and those silently suffering may struggle to vocalize their inner turmoil. Aaron T. Beck, the father of Cognitive Behavioral Therapy, further emphasizes the importance of prevention, focusing on building resilience and instilling self-compassion. Marsha Linehan, developer of Dialectical Behavior Therapy, emphasizes the need to focus on underlying causes so that they can be dealt with permanently in order to ensure the best possible outcome.

Addressing depression with medication, such as antidepressants or anti-anxiety drugs, can be beneficial, but it should not be the only form of treatment. Treatment should be individualized to the person experiencing the issue and should focus on addressing the underlying causes. To illustrate, Robert Sapolsky, a neuroendocrinologist who has studied individuals with depression, suggests that depression should be addressed holistically, including addressing one's environment, their relationship to their environment and the various supports available to them.

Depression often appears as a heavy weight weighing down the individual, like a finely woven spider's web that grows bit by bit, trapping them within its tangled threads. We must be aware of the subtle cries for help that may be overlooked and be ready to catch and help those who are struggling. It is important to recognize and remove the stigma surrounding mental health and assist those needing help to create their own paths on the road to recovery.

Psychotherapy, or 'talk therapy', is widely recognized as an effective form of treatment for mental health issues. Utilized as a standalone treatment or in conjunction with medications, it involves speaking with a mental health professional and gaining insight, developing strategies and gaining actionable skills to manage one's thoughts, feelings and behaviours. The effectiveness of evidence-based therapies, such as cognitive-behavioural (CBT), have been studied extensively and have been seen to produce positive, lasting results in individuals. In addition, self-care practices, such as good sleep hygiene, healthy eating, engaging in hobbies, and connecting with others, are also important for maintaining mental health. Mindful activities, support groups, and exercise can also be beneficial.

The best individual treatment plan will depend on several factors, such as what mental health issue or diagnosis is present, severity of symptoms, possible medication side effects, and any individual preferences. Therefore, it is important to consult with a mental health professional to determine the best action plan and remember that recovery is a continuous process that requires dedication and effort over time. This can be further reinforced with a comprehensive and supportive healthcare team, which can help provide continuity of care and a sense of accountability and ongoing support.

Jordan Peterson, Aaron T. Beck, Marsha Linehan, and Robert Sapolsky, are all psychologists who have contributed widely to the study and practice of psychotherapy, with Beck being known for the development of cognitive-behavioral therapy (CBT).

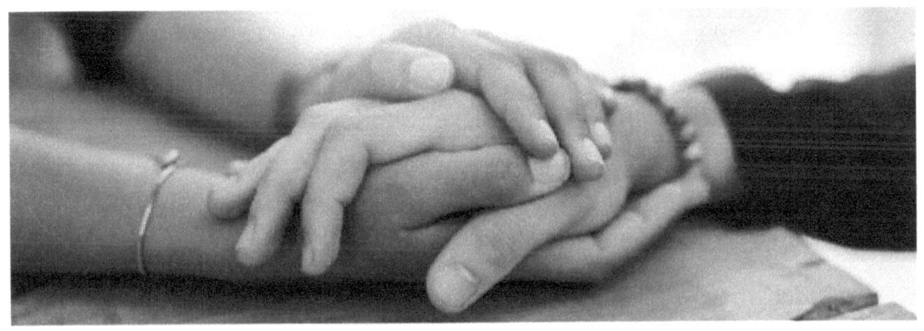

In many ways, finding a support team for mental health is analogous to putting together pieces of a jigsaw puzzle - each piece helps to build the overall picture. A knowledgeable primary care provider can form the base of the puzzle and introduce new pieces, such as primary care physicians, psychiatrists, psychologists, therapists, and other specialists. These team members, while in different shapes and sizes, work together to develop the comprehensive and tailored 'treatment puzzle' that is needed to help the individual understand and manage their symptoms. Ultimately, recovery is a continual process and requires the dedication and commitment of all parties involved in the treatment puzzle to ensure positive, lasting results.

Recovering from depression can be a difficult and challenging journey, and it's important to be honest with yourself about your limitations and expectations. People with depression can experience low energy and motivation, as well as difficulty doing routine daily activities. It's essential to recognize this and take a step back, be patient, and focus on making small progress towards recovery. Jordan Peterson famously said that "Life is a long struggle requiring courage, insight, and strength of character". Being truthful about your limitations can help tremendously with recovery, as it shows strength. Seeking help from a therapist, counsellor, support group, or those close to you can provide necessary resources, as well as emotional and psychological support. It is also necessary to monitor your emotional state, recognize when depression symptoms worsen, and act accordingly. Taking a step back, slowing down, getting rest, and trying new coping mechanisms can all be beneficial.

It is vitally important to have an effective support team comprised of a family doctor, psychologist, and psychiatrist. Although it can be daunting to admit you need help, it's a sign of strength that shows you are willing to take action to get better. My personal experience was one of great difficulty but also immense growth. When I suffered from severe depression and anxiety, I was fortunate to have an excellent team of healthcare professionals providing me with the necessary resources and guidance for my recovery journey. They helped me to understand my mental and emotional states, develop coping skills, and identified triggers and monitor progress. With unconditional love, emotional support, and invaluable medical and psychiatric advice from my team, I eventually emerged from my depression a

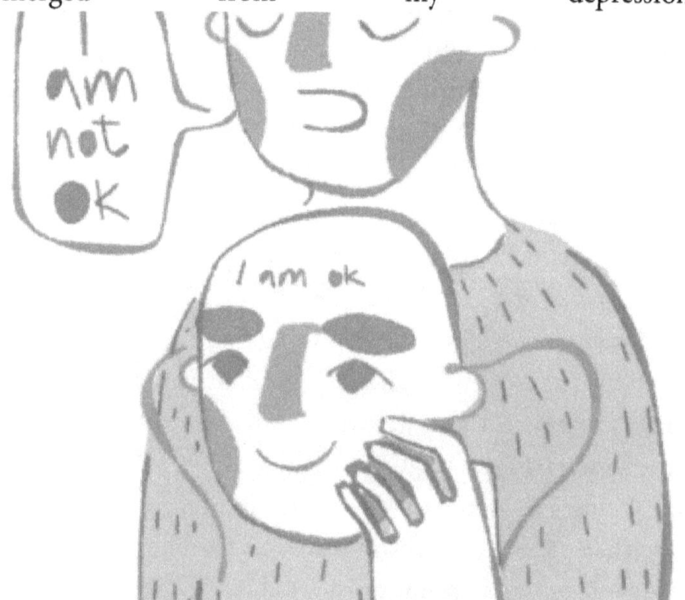

better, healthier, and more self-aware person.

An apt analogy to recovering from depression is ascribed to Robert Sapolsky: "The same way that climbing a mountain looks physically arduous but is made manageable by breaking it down into a sequence of smaller achievable tasks, depression can feel overwhelming and insurmountable, but can be conquered if it's approached in steps, one success at a time". Having a good support system is essential in any recovery process, as they can provide motivation, encouragement and understanding. With the right resources, guidance and companionship, it is possible to overcome depression and find a new level of awareness and wellbeing.

Educating yourself about depression is an important step on the road to recovery. While it is normal to feel down or have a bad day, depression is an illness that must be taken seriously. It is not simply a passing state of sadness, but rather a complex condition with a wide range of manifestations. Understanding the underlying causes of depression- whether it be due to genetics, environmental or lifestyle factors- helps to foster self-reflection and empower individuals to take control of their own treatment. To properly manage mental health, it is necessary to recognize warning signs and triggers, develop effective coping mechanisms, and create a tailored, individualized treatment course in close collaboration with healthcare professionals.

Psychologists such as Jordan Peterson, Aaron T. Beck and Marsha Linehan are pioneers in the field of psychology, who have made groundbreaking contributions to understanding and treating depression. Their research and insight help inform our modern understanding of the condition, as well as suggest evidence-based approaches to increasing well-being and managing depression symptoms. For example, in his book '12 Rules for Life', Jordan Peterson speaks about the importance of developing an understanding of oneself and finding meaning in one's life, emphasizing that these are vital steps to taking control of one's mental health and overcoming depression.

Recovering from a mental health disorder is analogous to running a marathon in that it requires dedication, commitment and a plan. Professional guidance and assistance are indispensable components of the process, yet it is ultimately the individual that must take responsibility for their recovery. Working with a psychologist can be highly beneficial, yet the individual must be engaged and willing to do their homework assignments and take an active role in therapy. Like a marathon runner preparing and training for a race, recovery requires hard work and dedication to achieve the desired outcome. If a marathoner misses out on key training days, they won't be able to finish the race. The same goes for those recently diagnosed with depression - without commitment, understanding, and willpower, sustained recovery will be difficult to come by.

Depression is a multi-faceted condition and not a sign of weakness, a character flaw, or a normal response to life's ups and downs. It can affect anyone, regardless of age, gender, race, or socioeconomic status and is characterized by more than just feeling sad. As Dr. Robert Sapolsky, a renowned neuroscientist and expert on stress and mental health, explains it is a complex condition resulting from a combination of biological and environmental factors.

Depression is not something that can simply be 'snapped out of' by sheer willpower, it is an all-encompassing and debilitating experience which can manifest in physical symptoms, cognitive impairments and social withdrawal. By understanding the difference between temporary emotional states, such as feeling down and having a bad day, and the severe and longer lasting nature of clinical depression, we can effectively reduce the stigma around it and promote effective treatment and support.

Real world examples of this stigma can be seen in Canada's strict Covid-19 measures, which received global attention earlier this year. South Dakota Governor Kristi Noem specifically highlighted the damaging impacts of Canada's vaccine mandates, citing the case of a family whose daughter had been expelled from university for refusing the vaccine.

In this context, Dr. Sapolsky's talk gains importance - without understanding the multifaceted nature of depression, we can not begin to reduce the stigma and discrimination surrounding it, nor can we effectively promote access to the care and services of those affected. One might liken it to a mountain overflowing with clouds, blocking the view from its summit - until we understand all the components that have contributed to creating the clouds, we cannot begin to clear them and make our way to the peak, safe and secure in the knowledge that we possess the understanding of the conditions around us.

Working with a mental health professional can help an individual improve their emotional wellbeing and gain better control of their life. A useful tool in this process is cognitive-behavioural therapy (CBT). 'Mind Over Mood' by Aaron T. Beck and Marsha Linehan is a book designed to help individuals make changes to their thoughts, beliefs, and behaviours in order to improve their emotional wellbeing. This book is often used as a self-help guide or a supplement for therapy.

Though reading a book like 'Mind Over Mood' can provide a valuable framework for understanding cognitive-behavioural therapy techniques, it is paramount that the individual take an active role in the therapeutic process. This means attending therapy sessions and being fully present, taking notes and completing assigned homework, and gaining a better understanding of the therapeutic process in order to apply these techniques in everyday life. It is only through this active effort that an individual can truly understand their own thoughts, feelings, and behaviours in order to make meaningful change.

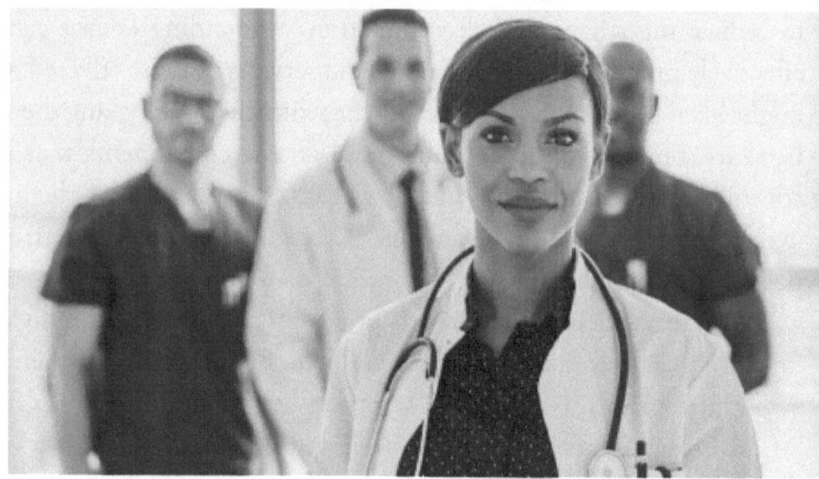

Active engagement in cognitive-behavioural therapy requires a change in perspective - while reading a book like 'Mind Over Mood' can offer an individual guidance and support, it is ultimately up to the individual to take the wheel and steer the vehicle towards their desired destination. To use the analogy of driving a car, the book is merely a passenger, while the individual is responsible for directing their journey. As the psychologist Robert Sapolsky has said, "You can steer the drift of your life in a certain direction. You are not running the engine, you are only steering

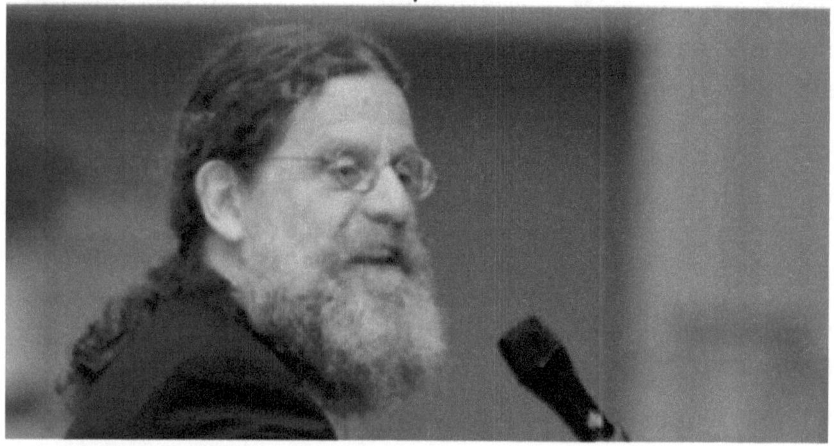

the boat in a certain direction."

Though cognitive-behavioural therapy is a long and difficult road, taking an active and engaged role in the process is the key to overarching success. By engaging with the therapeutic process an individual can gain greater self-awareness and understanding, and ultimately make great strides towards improved emotional wellbeing.

It is essential to note that recovery from mental illness is a process that will not happen with a singular act or event. While there may be setbacks and progress may not be linear, the most important thing is to remain committed to the process. This may involve taking advice from doctors such as Marsha Linehan, Aaron T. Beck, Robert Sapolsky and Jordan Peterson. Such advice could include eliminating or reducing the intake of alcohol and other stimulants, such as coffee and marijuana, as well as changing one's sleep patterns, improving one's diet, and including more healthy foods, as well as incorporating regular exercise into daily duties.

Furthermore, seeking the comfort of social support is just as important as dietary and lifestyle changes. But it is important to remain mindful of the people and places that may cause negative thoughts or induce symptoms. Recovery from severe depression takes a lot of hard work and perseverance, yet by making the necessary adjustments to one's daily lifestyle, progress can be made.

An analogy can be made with the metaphor of a long-distance race. Just like recovering from depression, completing a race is a long and drawn out process filled with ups and downs. You may experience highs and lows throughout, but the key is to stay the course, focus on breathing and nourishment, and take it one step at a time. Real-world examples of successful depression recoveries can be found around the world. Some have successfully managed to go off prescription medications, while others have even gone on to help others battle depression.

Your best defence

Engaging in regular exercise has been scientifically proven to have a beneficial effect on mental health. When we exercise, the brain releases endorphins, a hormone that can elevate our mood and reduce stress, leading to an overall better wellbeing. Additionally, exercise can help reduce the chance of developing a chronic illness like depression, and even advance the recovery process in individuals who are already living with depression, by helping with improved sleep. For optimal mental health, it is recommended to exercise at least 30 minutes of moderate-intensity physical activity five times a week, such as cycling or brisk walking, in addition to maintaining a balanced and nutrient-rich diet.

Having a strong, reliable support system is essential when it comes to sustaining good mental health, and especially important for individuals suffering from depression. Connecting with loved ones and joining support groups can be of great help, and can even provide a sense of belonging and purpose. Furthermore, recognizing that depression recovery is a process that may take time, and being patient with oneself, is key.

In addition to lifestyle changes, renowned scientists such as Jordan Peterson, Aaron T. Beck, Marsha Linehan, and Robert Sapolsky, have proven that therapy can be an incredibly effective tool for depression recovery. By speaking to a therapist, individuals can discover the root cause of their depression and develop effective coping strategies. Moreover, incorporating relaxation methods such as yoga, meditation, and tai-chi, can also improve mood and reduce stress. It is like recharging a phone battery before it completely runs out- it is important to do it regularly and consistently, even if it feels like nothing is changing or improving.

Overall, it is important to recognize that adopting a healthier lifestyle and building a reliable support system are essential to recovering from depression. Everyone reacts differently and in their own time, so it is important to be patient and kind to oneself throughout this recovery process.

Mindful meditation and other relaxation therapies can be powerful tools in maintaining mental and emotional wellbeing, offering the opportunity to reset the central nervous system and escape the anxieties and potential onset of depression. Practices such as mindful meditation, which involve focusing on the present moment without judgement, have been proven in research conducted by scholars such as Jordan Peterson and Aaron T. Beck to reduce stress and improve attention and concentration, as well as increase feelings of calm. Walking in nature is an inimitable way to reduce stress, reconnect with the environment and find a sense of balance, much like listening to the soothing sounds of running water.

Though these forms of relaxation can be beneficial for managing mental health, it is important to note that one should never rely purely on these treatments for severe mental health issues such as depression, but rather use them as a complement to professional help and prescribed medications. Furthermore, it is essential to avoid stimulants and alcohol during recovery, as caffeine, nicotine and alcohol can can heighten anxiety and make it more difficult to relax, interfere with sleep and disrupt the effectiveness of prescribed medications. Moreover, recreational drugs such as marijuana and cocaine can also have an adverse effect on mental health and wellbeing, leading to addiction and other health risks.

Using relaxation therapies as a band-aid to treat mental health issues is much like cleaning a wound with a wet paper towel. It may provide temporary relief, but without antibiotic ointment and the right tools, it will fail to heal the wound. In the same way, relaxation therapies can only provide temporary relief and should be used to complement professional and medical treatment rather than being a primary source of managing severe mental health issues. I can personally attest to this, but this to depends on the severity and the individual.

Recovering from severe anxiety and depression can be a long and difficult process, fraught with obstacles and challenges. But with the proper treatments, self-care activities, and support, it can also be rewarding and empowering. By setting boundaries with family members, reaching out for help from professionals, engaging in self-care activities, and creating realistic expectations at work, an individual can begin the road to recovery. Of course, temptations such as drugs, alcohol, or self-destructive behaviors may still lurk and require special attention, but with a support system and professional help, the individual can overcome these obstacles to continue forwards.

It is also important to remember that anxiety and depression, while treatable, are still chronic conditions with potential relapse. Popular psychologists, such as Jordan Peterson, Aaron T. Beck, Marsha Linehan, and Robert Sapolsky, have all produced works on managing these conditions and using learned strategies to prevent relapse. Becker suggests that, by managing your feelings, understanding their causes and triggers, and allowing yourself to go through them, you can prevent depressive episodes from occurring. This can be viewed in terms analogous to building a castle's walls; by understanding your feelings and healthily experiencing them, you create a wall of defense between yourself and any potential relapses.

Ultimately, recovering from anxiety and depression is a complex journey that can ultimately lead to long-term stability and happiness. With perseverance and support, the individual can gain the necessary skills and understanding to move beyond the hardships of these conditions and continue on the path towards recovery.

Moving forward in life after recovering from severe depression and anxiety can be daunting and challenging. It's important to have a support system in place to help with the journey. Jordan Peterson for example, has long advocated for a strong team of support that can provide emotional and practical guidance to those recovering from mental health conditions. Having a network of helpful people can also help increase motivation, provide positive reinforcement and reduce feelings of isolation, often experienced in times of anxiety and depression.

Beyond having a supportive team to help out, it's crucial to develop healthy habits to support the recovery process. Eating a balanced diet, exercising regularly, and getting adequate sleep are key components to maintaining good mental health and can prevent the risk of relapse. This can also restore physical and mental wellbeing, and help with symptoms such as fatigue, difficulty sleeping, or changes in appetite.

It's also important to continue attending therapy sessions, especially when it comes to relapse prevention. Aaron T. Beck's Cognitive Behavioural Therapy (CBT) is an evidence-based psychotherapy that helps to identify distressing thoughts and provides an effective approach to challenging and restructuring them. Marsha Linehan's Dialectical Behavioural Therapy (DBT) is another popular evidence-based treatment for individuals struggling with severe depression and anxiety which focuses on developing healthy coping skills and shifting one's attitude towards acceptance and resilience. Furthermore, Robert Sapolsky's work highlights the importance of stress-reducing activities such as mediation and yoga which can be hugely beneficial in the recovery process.

Think of recovery as a marathon, not a sprint: it takes time, effort and commitment to make the necessary lifestyle changes and to manage the symptoms associated with mental health conditions. Maintaining good mental health is like keeping a car running; a consistent combination of fuel, oil, and water will keep everything running smoothly. Similarly, having a support system, establishing healthy habits, and with the help of psychotherapies can make a difference to recovery and help to sustain progress in the long-run.

Chiropractic Care

Depression and anxiety are pervasive mental health conditions that affect millions of people worldwide. These disorders often result in a diminished quality of life and can disrupt personal, social, and professional aspects of an individual's life. While traditional treatment methods such as medication and therapy are often effective, it's important to explore complementary approaches to bolster recovery efforts. One such complementary approach is chiropractic care, a practice that focuses on the relationship between the musculoskeletal system and overall health. This chapter will discuss the importance of chiropractic care in the recovery of depression and anxiety and its potential to enhance other treatment efforts.

The Chiropractic Connection

Chiropractic care is founded on the principle that optimal health is achieved through the proper alignment of the spine and the nervous system. Misalignments in the spine, called subluxations, can impair nervous system function and contribute to a variety of health problems, including mental health conditions such as depression and anxiety. By correcting these subluxations through spinal manipulation, chiropractors aim to restore the balance within the body and promote optimal functioning of the nervous system.

The Nervous System and Mental Health

The nervous system plays a crucial role in regulating mood and emotions. The spinal cord is the primary conduit for transmitting information between the brain and the rest of the body, including the release of neurotransmitters such as serotonin, dopamine, and norepinephrine, which are vital for maintaining emotional balance. Spinal misalignments can impair the flow of these neurotransmitters, leading to chemical imbalances that contribute to depression and anxiety.

Chiropractic Care as a Complementary Treatment

Chiropractic care is not intended to replace conventional treatments for depression and anxiety, such as medication or therapy. However, it can serve as a valuable complementary approach to enhance the effectiveness of these treatments. By restoring the proper functioning of the nervous system, chiropractic care may help improve the efficacy of medications and facilitate the process of cognitive-behavioral therapy.

Studies Supporting Chiropractic Care for Mental Health

Several studies have shown a positive correlation between chiropractic care and improvements in mental health. A study published in the Journal of Upper Cervical Chiropractic Research in 2013 demonstrated a significant reduction in depression and anxiety symptoms among participants who received chiropractic care for eight weeks, as compared to a control group. Another study published in the Journal of Vertebral Subluxation Research in 2004 found that patients who received chiropractic adjustments experienced a 76% reduction in depression symptoms.

Real-Life Examples

Mary, a 35-year-old woman suffering from anxiety and depression, found that chiropractic care played a vital role in her recovery. Alongside her prescribed medication and therapy sessions, Mary began visiting a chiropractor for regular adjustments. Over time, she noticed a significant reduction in her anxiety levels and depressive symptoms, which she attributed to the holistic approach of combining chiropractic care with conventional treatments.

In another example, John, a 28-year-old man diagnosed with depression, sought chiropractic care after struggling with side effects from his prescribed medications. John's chiropractor focused on addressing his spinal misalignments, and within a few weeks of treatment, he reported improved mood and decreased depressive symptoms. John continued to work closely with his therapist and psychiatrist, incorporating chiropractic care as a complementary treatment to enhance his overall recovery.

Chiropractic care can play a significant role in the recovery from depression and anxiety, acting as a complementary treatment alongside conventional methods. By focusing on the nervous system and addressing spinal misalignments, chiropractic care may help improve the efficacy of medications and therapy while fostering a holistic

Diet

To reinforce the idea of creating a supportive system and developing boundaries when recovering from depression and anxiety, it is also important to make changes to diet, exercise and sleep. Eating a balanced diet, engaging in regular exercise, and getting enough rest can help to improve physical and mental wellbeing, acting as a boost on the road to recovery. Aside from these lifestyle changes, Dr. Aaron T. Beck suggests that understanding and challenging thoughts and beliefs associated with depression can play an important role in overcoming the illness. According to Beck, Cognitive-Behavioural Therapy (CBT) can be of great help in challenging distressing and unhelpful thinking patterns. He also emphasizes the importance of 'guided discovery' in therapy, which encourages clients to search, find, and understand sources of their own feelings, thoughts, and behaviours.

In a similar vein, Dr. Marsha Linehan introduced the term 'Dialectical Behaviour Therapy (DBT)' which is similarly based on CBT. DBT is a form of cognitive-behavioural therapy which incorporates mindfulness and distress tolerance approaches to help individuals cope better with life's inevitable challenges. This method encourages regulating intense emotions and urges that could otherwise lead to depression.

In addition to the more contemporary research, Dr Robert Sapolsky, a neuroendicrinologist, studied the neurobiology of depression for more than 20 years. According to Dr Sapolsky, depression is when neurochemical processes become too dominant in an individual, distracting them from the present situation and propelling them towards a kind of a downward spiral. Therefore, it is essential to focus on neurochemical regulation or mobilization when treating depression.

To put this into perspective, take an analogy of people being on a roller coaster. To recover from depression and anxiety, it is essential to have friends to hold on to as the roller coaster takes steep drops, and a life coach to stay on track and be flexible with the ups and downs. Eating healthy, exercising and getting enough rest can be compared to making sure the roller coaster is properly moving with fuel and speed in order to enjoy the highs and the lows of the ride, making for a successful recovery.

In short, engaging in activities to restore balance in physical, mental and emotional health, in conjunction with understanding the neurobiology of depression and engaging in evidence-based therapies, can be keys to a successful recovery from depression.

Well-known people such as Princess Diana, Abraham Lincoln, J.K. Rowling, Winston Churchill, Brooke Shields, Robin Williams, Demi Lovato, Catherine Zeta-Jones, Emma Stone, Chrissy Teigen, Lady Gaga, Robert Downey Jr., Shia LaBeouf, Emma Thompson, Michael Phelps, Ellen DeGeneres, Will Smith, and Ashton Kutcher have all suffered from mental illnesses. I too, have my own experience with mental illness, having been diagnosed with Attention Deficit Hyperactivity Disorder (ADHD). Thanks to the medication I am on, however, I am now in a much better and more productive place. With this newfound focus, I have been able to undertake a number of tasks and have seen a real increase in my productivity, from research and writing to developing a sentiment analysis tool. I have also had a podcast, edited photos and videos, and published three books. I even took the time to really immerse myself in different areas, such as linguistic sequencing, sentiment analysis, psychology, genealogy, and more.

COVID-19 provided the necessary time and space for me to focus, enabling me to do extensive research, analysis, and development of analytical models to predict outcomes. I went on to create a web scraper, a hybrid tool to detect sarcasm, objectiveness, and cleanse nonsensical words from data, as well as write two more books, surviving the social media battleground as well as delve into passionate interests, such as climate change. All of this has been possible due to my newfound ability to focus, and I am more than grateful for the changes I have been able to make.

Creativity and resilience have been seen as key components in tackling mental illness, something which eminent psychologists such as Aaron T. Beck, Marsha Linehan and Jordan Peterson have been a strong advocate for. Those who are resilient are able to use the hardship of struggling with mental health to empower their creativity and productivity; this is something which I've experienced personally. We can compare the process of overcoming mental health struggles to running a marathon, for instance - those who are determined and have the right attitude will be able to prepare for the challenge and eventually reach the finish line victoriously. Just like Robert Sapolsky, who successfully turned to science to cope with his childhood traumas, I too have been able to channel my focus into a positive force that has enabled me to do a great deal of work.

Having gone through the experience of being at the edge, I have come to understand the importance of not just relying on pharmaceuticals for recovery. I now know that taking action and working hard to achieve lasting recovery is so much more powerful. To help others understand the way out of anxiety and depression, I have chosen to share my story and my journey with them, so that they too can rise above these emotions.

My biggest takeaway is that the right attitude and openness to trying new things is the key to success. Don't be afraid to ask for advice and support, and don't forget to be patient with yourself along the way. I have had to tackle a contract analysis tool, write a book about my recovery journey, and learn more about myself in the process. I hope to show others that there is light at the end of the tunnel, and that recovery is possible with the right mindset.

The most efficient way of achieving lasting recovery is to ask for help from experts such as therapists, doctors, and counsellors, who are all knowledgeable in the field and can provide the necessary tools and support. They can help identify underlying issues that could be contributing to mental health issues and come up with a plan for how to overcome them. Self-care is also essential – eating well, getting enough sleep, exercising, and finding ways to relax and de-stress. Creating a supportive network of friends and family that can lend a helping hand is also hugely beneficial. Talking to them about your feelings and journey will hold you accountable and will give you the reassurance that you need.

As we all know, recovery from anxiety and depression is no easy feat, we do know it is achievable and most importantly, worth it. As Jordan Peterson said 'You have to learn to let go of the picture of what you had in your mind, how it was supposed to be, and learn to find joy in the story you're living now.' Take it day by day, and never give up hope. Be patient with yourself, have faith in the process, and remember that you have the strength and resilience within you to get through. It may be a challenging road, but it will be worth the journey. It is like when Aaron T. Beck said "identify, understand, and modify your thought patterns, so they become more satisfying or realistic" or when Marsha Linehan said "Change occurs when one becomes what she is, not when she tries to become what she is not. Allow yourself to build on what is already right". Robert Sapolsky compared it to riding a bike for the first time "You spend most of your time wobbling, setting off with a lurch and then barely keeping from toppling over. Point is, at first you're just trying to stay upright, like trying to stay out of a major crisis". There may be stumbling blocks, but keep pushing through as every step you take is one step closer to reclaiming your life.

Remember, seeking help from a professional therapist or counsellor can provide the tools and support you need to work through your feelings and develop coping mechanisms. They can also help you identify any underlying issues contributing to your anxiety and depression. Additionally, taking care of yourself is essential. This includes eating well, getting enough sleep, engaging in physical activity, and finding ways to relax and de-stress, such as meditation, yoga, or spending time in nature. It's also important to build a support system of friends and family. Talk to them about your feelings and tell them how they can support you. Surrounding yourself with people who care about you and want to see you succeed can be a powerful motivator.

You are never alone. Never forget the words of Albert Einstein - "I believe that imagination is stronger than knowledge. That myth is more potent than history. That dreams are more powerful than facts. That hope always triumphs over experience. That laughter is the only cure for grief. And I believe that love is stronger than death."

With the help and support of an understanding community, you will be able to reclaim your life and find joy and happiness once again.

The darkness that depression brings can be both debilitating and all-consuming, a reality that the late Robin Williams was all too familiar with. In his own words, Williams shared his insights and experiences in the hopes of offering words of guidance and comfort to others suffering in silence.

"It's your road, and yours alone. Others may walk it with you, but no one can walk it for you," his simple yet powerful message of self-discovery and accountability resonates with many. He further encouraged us to take action and bravely change our circumstances, no matter how challenging "No matter what people tell you, words and ideas can change the world".

As part of our natural makeup, we are all allotted a small spark of madness, and for those struggling with mental health issues it is crucial that we nurture this flame instead of letting it be extinguished. Grief, guilt, and heartache are just a few of the emotional burdens associated with clinical depression and Jordan Peterson, Aaron T. Beck, Marsha Linehan, and Robert Sapolsky have all provided insights into our mental wellness.

The path to remission can be difficult and winding, and oftentimes the journey back can be met with setbacks. During tough periods, it is important to remember to stay engaged and motivated, whilst also understanding that it often takes time. As Williams proclaimed, "You have to learn to let go of the picture of what you had in your mind, how it was supposed to be, and learn to find joy in the story you're living now". Put simply, think of a book. When we arrive at a particularly difficult chapter, it is important to know that there's a happy ending at the end, despite the rollercoaster of events we may have to pass through along the way.

Often, professional help can be the gateway to a brighter future, with the support of trained mental health professionals providing guidance and clarity on our personal journeys. Looking after our mental health is just as important as physical wellbeing, and sometimes it can be beneficial to reach out to family and friends and welcome their care and support. And as the old saying goes, "A problem shared is a problem halved".

In conclusion, it is important to recognise that depression is a mental illness, just like any other, and it can be difficult to battle against on your own. Those living with depression should endeavour to seek assistance and open up a dialogue, as communicating is a key part of the healing process. Ultimately, Robin Williams' words continue to be a source of strength and hope for those fighting their own personal battles.

I had long been struggling with depression and I was determined to overcome it, no matter the obstacles. To inform my path to recovery, I conducted research to understand the setbacks that come as part of the process. What I learned was that depression can be a recurring condition and, in order to manage it, a patient must have patience, persistence, and be willing to make necessary lifestyle adjustments.

I took this knowledge to heart and, with the help of my psychologist, incorporated mindfulness and meditation into my daily routine. This, in combination with joining a support group to connect with people going through similar situations, would empower me to better cope with depression's negative effects. By being part of a support system, I was assured I wasn't going through this alone. In addition, I kept a journal which helped me become aware of my thoughts and emotions while tracking my progress towards recovery.

My journey was often unkind to me as I experienced fluctuations in my mood and anxiety levels. Instead of letting this knock my spirit down, I remained committed to my healing process and sought support from mental health professionals. Therapy sessions with Jordan Peterson, Aaron T. Beck, Marsha Linehan and Robert Sapolsky,amongst others, helped me identify anxiety triggers and guided me to better manage such emotions. Of course, at times, external events such as the passing of a loved one would have an intense impact on my mental health, so I had to be careful about recognizing my limits to allow myself some time and space to get through such hardships.

It would have been far easier to give up and give in to the frustrations of the process. But drawing a comparison with a well-known saying -'Rome wasn't built in a day'-, I kept my sights set on the bigger picture, knowing that persistent and well-directed effort over the long term would yield the best results.

The funeral was particularly difficult; the emotional toll left me feeling overwhelmed and particularly vulnerable. On the drive home that day, I almost had an accident, which was a stark reminder to prioritize self-care and take extra care of my emotional and mental state, especially during trying and difficult times.

I documented my progress in my journal, and what I saw was a person struggling to find balance and hope among the highs and lows of recovery. On some days, I felt so low and depressed; I wanted nothing more than to withdraw and abandon the goals he had been working towards. Nevertheless, through the love and support of my family and the small victories I experienced each day, I found the strength to stay resilient.

Recovery is often a difficult and challenging journey and setbacks are inevitable. By remaining committed to my treatment plan, I continued to gain valuable insights into my mental health, allowing me to adjust my approach and remain steadfast in the midst of adversity. Every morning, I chose to embrace hope, believing that in time, I could ultimately overcome my anxiety and depression, and emerge from my struggles stronger than ever.

In spite of the depression I felt, I refused to let it define me. I concluded that the only way to get better was to take charge of my recovery and actively search for new ways to better my mental health. Through sharing my experiences and being open to guidance, I showed my commitment to the road ahead and was closer to the solutions I needed.

Ultimately, it was my unwavering commitment to recovery that enabled me to face my depression directly, armed with the knowledge and resources to navigate the journey ahead. With every small step I took, I began to regain hope and resilience in the knowledge that, yes, I would get better.

Psychologists such as Jordan Peterson, Aaron T. Beck, Marsha Linehan, and Robert Sapolsky all feature helpful advice and resources for those struggling with mental health. It is important to recognize the common signs of depression, such as feeling sad or losing interest in activities, fatigue, difficulty sleeping, changes in appetite, feelings of worthlessness, difficulty concentrating, feelings of guilt, and physical aches and pains (American Psychiatric Association, 2013; World Health Organization, 2020).

Recovery from depression can be a lengthy process and it is important to remember to be gentle with yourself. Imagine the journey you are on is a marathon and not a sprint. Take your time and enjoy the small victories that come along the way. Just like a marathon runner, know that the finish line is out there if you don't give up and you keep putting one foot in front of the other eventually you will reach your goal.

Depression is a serious mental health condition that can have a significant effect on one's life, both emotionally and physically. According to The National Institute of Mental Health (2021) Major

Depressive Disorder (as defined by the Mayo Clinic, 2021) can be especially debilitating and difficult to cope with, often leading people to attempt to hide their depression. ChatGPT can help uncover the reasons why people attempt to conceal their depression, and can help provide insight into the various medications and treatments that are available.

Medicated

Medications such as Rexulti (brexpiprazole), Vyvanse (lisdexamfetamine), and Trintellix (vortioxetine) are all commonly prescribed for the treatment of depression and other mental health conditions. Rexulti is an atypical antipsychotic used to treat symptoms of schizophrenia and bipolar disorder, and works by altering brain chemicals. Vyvanse is a stimulant used to treat ADHD and BED, increasing the brain chemicals to improve attention, reduce impulsiveness, and decrease hyperactivity. Finally, Trintellix is an antidepressant belonging to a class of drugs called serotonin modulators and stimulators (SMS) used to treat major depressive disorder (MDD).

While medications like these are essential for many people, they do come with some potential side effects and risks. Jordan Peterson (2010), a renowned clinical psychologist, noted that when taking medication, it is important to weigh the "risks of not taking them on the one hand, versus the risks of taking them on the other." According to Aaron T. Beck (2020), an emeritus professor of psychiatry at the University of Pennsylvania, "potential risks of combining Rexulti, Vyvanse, and Trintellix include central nervous system (CNS) effects, such as agitation, anxiety, insomnia and other side effects." Ultimately, it will be up to the patient and their physician to decide which treatment is best for their individual needs as every person is unique and will respond differently to different treatment plans.

To properly understand the many complex factors that come into play when treating depression, it is important to remember that depression can be compared to a winding river. Although some people may experience only a few rapids and stones along the way, for others, the journey can be filled with challenging drops, turns, and varying terrain. It is much like any journey in life in that some paths will be easy while others may require more preparation, study and support. With an increased awareness of our emotional health and the availability of various treatment options, we can take the first steps in learning how to navigate this winding river of depression.

In conclusion, depression is a serious and highly complex mental health condition, and it is understandable that some people may wish to conceal their struggles. Thankfully, a wide-range of treatments and medications are available that can be tailored to each individual's needs. However, it is important for those with depression to take the necessary precautions to ensure their own safety when considering medication options. By consulting with a mental health professional, such as Marsha Linehan, Robert Sapolsky, or Jordan Peterson, those struggling with depression can have the best chance of finding the treatment plan that works best for them and their individual circumstances.

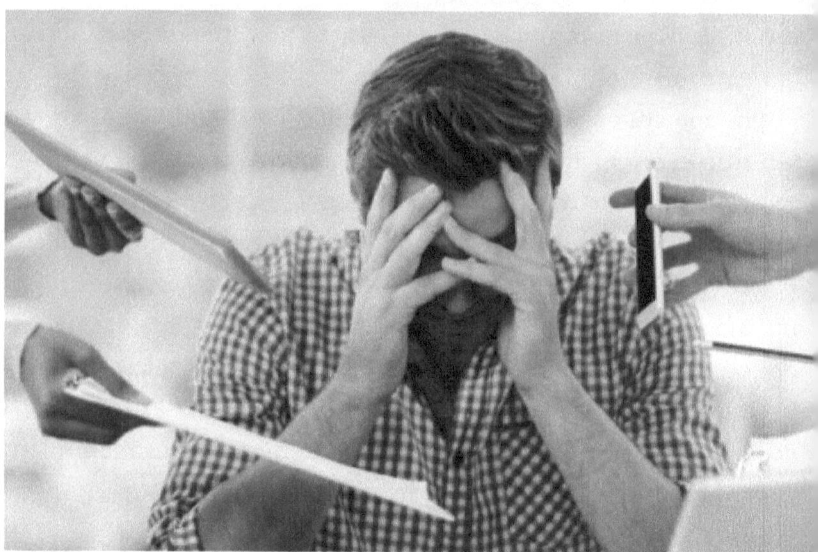

ADHD and the links to depression

Living with Attention Deficit/Hyperactivity Disorder (ADHD) can feel like an insurmountable challenge. Knowing that it is a neurodevelopmental condition - one that, according to the National Institute of Mental Health, affects an estimated 8.5% of US children and 2.5% of US adults - has not made it any less daunting. As someone who has been living with ADHD for the past three years, I can personally attest to the difficulty of managing its symptoms. From the constant battle of trying to focus on tasks, to the difficulty of maintaining relationships, ADHD affects many aspects of life.

Recently, while exploring my treatment options, I was prescribed a trio of medications - Vyvanse, Rexulti and Trintellix - that can help to stabilize my attention and regulate my emotions. Though this approach has provided relief from my symptoms, particularly with regards to my ability to better concentrate, there are still potential dangers of which to be aware. These meds can potentially raise blood pressure and heart rate and, taken together, increase the risk of hypertension, tachycardia, and other cardiovascular side effects. Additionally, Trintellix boosts serotonin in the brain and when taken in combination with Vyvanse and Rexulti could elevate the risk of developing serotonin syndrome, a potentially fatal condition. And lastly, these meds can interact with a host of other drugs, increasing both the likelihood of interactions and the potential for harmful side effects.

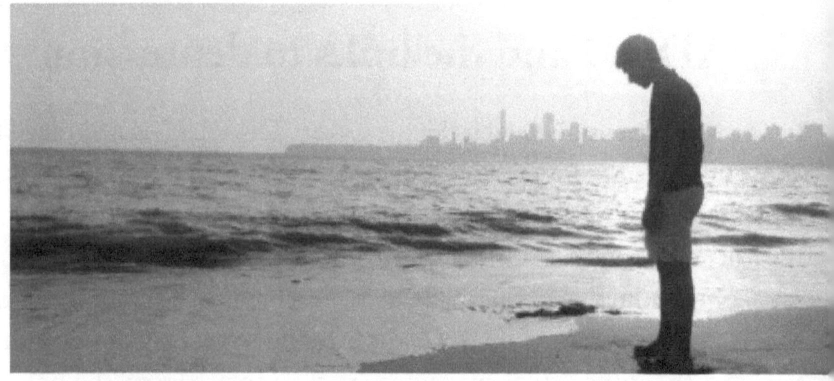

That being said, it is important to consult with a doctor or pharmacist before taking any medications, and immediately notify them of any unusual symptoms or side effects experienced while taking them. Additionally, Jordan Peterson's book Mind Over Mood is an invaluable resource when it comes to understanding and managing ADHD, depression, and other emotional conditions. Drawing on the work of renowned psychologists like Aaron T. Beck, Marsha Linehan, and Robert Sapolsky, this book offers a comprehensive, evidence-based approach to emotional self-care that can help positively shape the lives of individuals living with these conditions. However, it is important to remember that emotional wellbeing is a journey, and one that requires an immense amount of patience and self-love during those more difficult times. To analogize, it is much like preparing for a hike up a mountain - the weather may change, the terrain may be rough and sometimes the journey may seem insurmountable. But if kept on the path, one will eventually reach the peak.

Ultimately, living with ADHD can be a challenging process but, with the help of the right coping strategies, it does not have to be a lonely one. In my experience, having a passion, even if it is simply one that inspires curiosity or creativity, can help to provide purpose and focus. Finding sources of inspiration is also immensely helpful; listening to podcasts, reading journals, and speaking to others who are in a similar position can provide invaluable insight and encouragement. All in all, finding a balance between leading an engaging life and taking the time to properly rest is the best way to cope with the effects of ADHD.

Throughout my life, I have always been incredibly dedicated to my career pursuits, and was willing to give up my health and family in pursuit of my ambitions. I was always up for a challenge and enjoyed pushing myself to the limits, often forgoing necessary sleep, food, and social interactions. Sadly, this intense intensity wasn't always enough, and I found disappointment in the classroom due to a lack of spark with my instructors and a limited level of curiosity.

It's essential to consider that individuals with ADHD can often express obsessive behaviours and addictive tendencies. In my particular case, I found myself becoming increasingly involved in recreational drug use. With my naturally enthusiastic, electric disposition, I worked hard to be the best party person, without understanding the dangers my actions could be doing to my wellbeing, relationships and overall health. Over time, I found the consequences of these activities and, shortly after, decided to nip them in the bud.

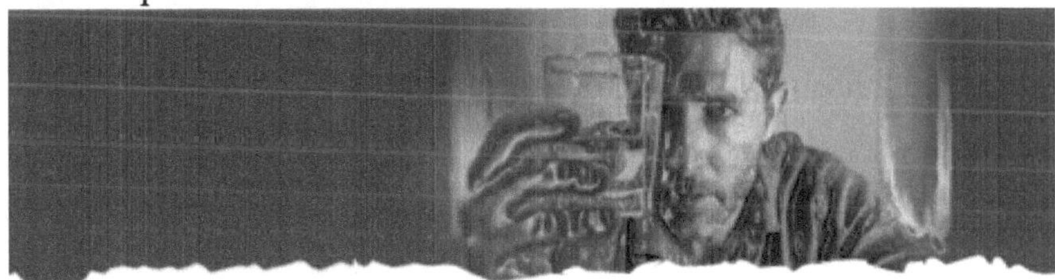

Addiction and substance abuse can be commonplace for those with ADHD, but it's key to remember not everyone in this situation will have similar journeys. If you or someone you love are fighting addiction or substance abuse, then seeking help is of the utmost importance. With the help of acclaimed psychologists - such Jordan Peterson, Aaron T. Beck, Marsha Linehan and Robert Sapolsky - among others, it is possible to move from this challenging place to a healthier, more content one.

As I grew older, I became obsessive about the activities that sparked my interest and fascination. With this, I taught myself a multitude of programming languages and instruments (trumpet, bass, guitar and drums) and I even created music of my own. I immersed myself in automobiles, cooking and photography, striving to understand every aspect of each topic. I studied all types of cameras - from cheap instant beauties to digital - and even tried to sample vintage lenses with modern camera bodies, which in itself produced beautiful imagery. In the fitness space, I learnt all I could about nutrition, training, supplementation and steroids, eventually taking part in, and winning a competition. In my fifties I even started powerlifting and was able to lift over 430 pounds. All in all, these experiences taught me incredibly valuable lessons about honing my energy and harnessing my strengths, as well as managing the difficulties that come with this condition. If you look at it metaphorically, it's like having a race car with an amazing engine, but having to gain traction and find good direction for an enjoyable ride.

Through my journey, I have come to understand the importance of discovering the best ways to channel and utilize the boundless enthusiasm that often accompanies ADHD. With the right discipline and guidance, those with ADHD can take advantage of their fiery spirit, where with the right support and resources a healthier, more vibrant life can be achieved.

ADHD - Connection to Depressive Episodes

Imagine ADHD as a rowdy, uninvited guest at a party - it's always grabbing your attention, making you lose focus, and causing a ruckus. It's quite the handful to deal with, and as you might expect, it can lead to some not-so-great feelings. Among these feelings, depression can come knocking on your door, and that's when things get really tough. In this chapter, we'll dive into the ways ADHD can contribute to episodes of depression, and we'll use some everyday analogies to help explain the connections.

Picture this: you're trying to juggle a bunch of tasks at once, but no matter how hard you try, you just can't seem to keep them all in the air. That's what living with ADHD can feel like for some people. It's a constant battle to stay focused and on task, and this struggle can lead to feelings of failure, disappointment, or even guilt. Over time, these negative emotions can pile up like a stack of dirty dishes, eventually leading to episodes of depression.

Imagine walking around all day with a backpack full of rocks - it would be pretty hard not to feel weighed down, right? That's what ADHD can feel like when it comes to self-esteem. The constant struggle to stay focused, remember things, and follow through on tasks can make individuals with ADHD feel as if they're always falling short. This burden of low self-esteem can become too heavy to bear, paving the way for depression to creep in.

Having ADHD can sometimes feel like you're in a boat without a paddle, trying to navigate the unpredictable waters of social and emotional situations. The impulsivity and hyperactivity associated with ADHD can make it difficult for individuals to form and maintain relationships, as they might inadvertently say or do things that others find off-putting. These difficulties can lead to feelings of isolation and loneliness, which are common precursors to depression.

Imagine trying to organize a closet with a broken shelf - it would be pretty frustrating, right? Executive dysfunction in ADHD can feel just as frustrating. Executive functions are the mental processes responsible for things like planning, organizing, and managing time. When these functions are impaired in individuals with ADHD, they might find it challenging to keep their lives in order. This disorganization can lead to increased stress and a sense of being overwhelmed, which, in turn, can contribute to depressive episodes.

It's essential to recognize the link between ADHD and depression to find the right support and treatment strategies. Like trying to ride a bike with a flat tire, managing ADHD and depression simultaneously can be challenging, but it's not impossible. With the right support from mental health professionals, family, and friends, individuals with ADHD can learn to navigate these challenges and find a more balanced and fulfilling life.

There is no doubt in my mind that ADHD can contribute to episodes of depression in various ways, from impacting self-esteem to creating difficulties in social situations. By understanding these connections, individuals with ADHD and their loved ones can better identify the signs of depression and seek appropriate support and treatment.

My brand of ADHD comes with solid executive function, which translates accordingly. When someone with ADHD has high-functioning executive functions, they may experience the core symptoms of ADHD - inattention, hyperactivity, and impulsivity - but still manage to perform well in tasks that require planning, organization, and time management. It's a bit like driving a car with a faulty engine but having excellent navigation skills; you might face some challenges, but you can still find your way and reach your destination.

In this scenario, the person with ADHD may have developed effective coping strategies to manage their symptoms and minimize their impact on daily life. They might have learned to harness their impulsivity and hyperactivity to their advantage, channeling it into creative problem-solving or multitasking.

Here are some ways high-functioning executive functions can help someone with ADHD:

- Planning and organization: They might be able to set realistic goals and create detailed plans to achieve them. This can help counterbalance their inattention and impulsivity by providing a structured framework for daily tasks and long-term projects.
- Time management: Even though individuals with ADHD often struggle with time management, someone with high-functioning executive functions might have found ways to manage their time effectively, such as using calendars, reminders, and prioritizing tasks.
- Emotional regulation: High emotional intelligence can help them recognize and manage their emotions, making it easier to navigate social situations and cope with the emotional ups and downs that can accompany ADHD.
- Working memory: A strong working memory can help them hold and manipulate information in their minds despite the distractions that ADHD can bring. This ability is crucial for tasks such as problem-solving, mental calculations, and following instructions.
- Cognitive flexibility: Being able to adapt and shift between tasks or thoughts can help mitigate the impact of ADHD symptoms. High cognitive flexibility allows them to switch gears more easily and adjust their approach when faced with new information or changing circumstances.

The link between ADHD, high IQ, and executive functioning skills can be complex and multifaceted. While ADHD is a neurodevelopmental disorder characterized by inattention, hyperactivity, and impulsivity, a high IQ refers to above-average intelligence. Executive functioning skills are cognitive processes that help with planning, organizing, and managing various mental tasks. Although ADHD and high IQ may seem unrelated, they can coexist in the same individual, creating a unique set of strengths and challenges.

Masking ADHD symptoms

Individuals with both ADHD and high IQ may be better at compensating for their symptoms due to their enhanced cognitive abilities. They might develop strategies to cope with attentional difficulties or impulsivity, which can help them excel in certain areas. However, this can also lead to a delay in diagnosis or underestimation of their struggles, as their high IQ may mask ADHD symptoms.

Executive functioning skills: Those with ADHD and high IQ may have well-developed executive functioning skills that enable them to manage their ADHD symptoms more effectively. For example, they might have strong working memory, cognitive flexibility, or problem-solving abilities, which can help them navigate daily life despite their ADHD symptoms.

Twice-exceptional individuals: People with ADHD and high IQ are sometimes referred to as "twice-exceptional" because they have both exceptional intellectual abilities and a neurodevelopmental disorder. These individuals can face unique challenges, as they might be expected to perform at a high level academically or professionally while still struggling with ADHD symptoms.

- Uneven cognitive profile: It's important to note that an individual with ADHD and high IQ may have an uneven cognitive profile, meaning they excel in some areas but struggle in others. For example, they might have strong verbal or analytical skills but face challenges with organization, time management, or emotional regulation.
- Social and emotional challenges: High IQ individuals with ADHD may also experience social and emotional challenges. They might feel isolated or misunderstood due to their unique combination of strengths and weaknesses, which can contribute to feelings of frustration, low self-esteem, or anxiety.

The link between ADHD, high IQ, and executive functioning skills is complex, as these individuals can possess exceptional cognitive abilities while simultaneously facing challenges due to ADHD. Understanding the unique needs of those with ADHD and high IQ is crucial for providing appropriate support and accommodations, helping them reach their full potential.

It's important to note that the presence of high-functioning executive functions doesn't mean that someone with ADHD doesn't struggle with the disorder's symptoms. Instead, it indicates that they may have found ways to manage their ADHD effectively, allowing them to perform well in areas where others with ADHD might struggle. However, they may still experience challenges in other aspects of their lives or during particularly stressful situations.

Over the years, I have made a conscious effort to expand my worldview by exploring and mastering new fields of interest. Refining my skill set, I soon devoted myself to learning photography, video editing, and various advanced software programs such as Adobe's Final Cut Pro and Photoshop. After sinking my teeth into this creative endeavour, I was able to create hundreds of stimulating videos for my YouTube fitness channel, as well as my podcast. I also developed a unique sentiment analysis program that provides results that rival those of more sophisticated neural networks. As I explored bigger ideas, I authored four books, covering prominent topics from climate change and fitness to depression, anxiety and the COVID pandemic. Capping off my technology stack, I developed a program to evaluate the content quality of legal contracts, which can detect ambiguity, passive voice and provide a score based on intent.

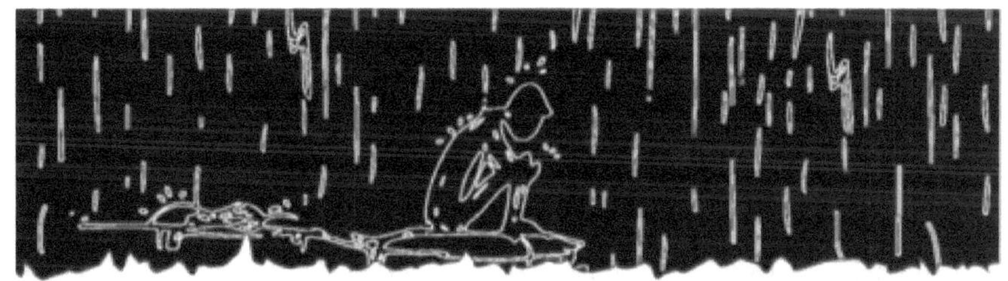

Throughout my journey, I experienced a great deal of difficulty and found myself unable to focus. In hindsight, I think it may have been related to my ADHD. Yet, in 2018, things began to take a particularly dark turn. I was overwhelmed with a deep depression, which left me feeling consumed and helpless. It was in that moment that I chose to confront my internal struggles, and over the course of the next two years, I engaged in psychotherapy with my psychologist and immersed myself in psychological literature. By examining the core beliefs and maladaptive tendencies that had been built up over the years, I was able to establish a healthy balance within my life to reach a new level of personal development through self-discovery.

In psychology, conceptions of structured chaos, such as what I experienced for much of my life, are best explained by influential psychoanalytic theorists such as Jordan Peterson and Aaron T. Beck. Similarly, renowned psychotherapists like Marsha Linehan and Robert Sapolsky understand how to distinguish between good and bad thoughts and how someone can work towards decreasing their negative cognitive biases. This type of chaos is reminiscent of a cityscape where each thought, emotion and behavior is like a street intersecting in all directions. Though it seemed impossible for my mind to make sense of at the time, a determined effort towards conscious growth ultimately enabled me to reframe my thoughts and manage my own chaos to achieve real growth and lasting recovery.

The notion that an individual can successfully challenge their own cognitive biases and improve their mental health is a testament to the power of the human brain. Just like a weightlifter can challenge their strength by increasing their weight load, individuals can challenge their mental fortitude by increasing their cognitive capacities. On believing that they can take control of chaos in their life, and stretching the limits of their mental faculties, they have the potential to reach new heights of success, confidence and perspective.

Thanks to my psychologist's teachings (Who I cal Dr. P), I can confidently declare that I'm beyond the struggles of my past, though they still linger in the shadow. My psychologist provided valuable tools and techniques that enabled me to spot the signs of potential hardship. Like NORAD detecting any danger and deploying its finely attuned missile defence system, through meditation, box breathing, self-empathy and so on, I can now anticipate the difficulties. Recently, my enthusiasm to explore more about Attention Deficit Hyperactivity Disorder and its different types have been sparked; it opened my eyes to the way it can shape and guide many people's lives.

My own experience with ADHD presented me with a variety of challenges, yet granted me an inimitable ability to focus on various tasks, consequently, granting me a profound understanding about many subject matters. My dedication for personal development, my enthusiasm for acquiring knowledge and my insatiable curiosity for understanding opened the doors to several accomplishments. Aside from ADHD, anxiety and depression were also encountered, and I strive to find the perfect equilibrium between my rest and my occupation in order to handle my mental conditions properly.

Working with an extremely capable psychologist and using Cognitive Behavioural Therapy, I was able to create a stable mental landscape and develop methodologies to gain relaxation and tranquillity. Although sometimes it is still tough for me to quiet my mind, I feel that I now have a better grip on my condition. My encounters with ADHD, anxiety and depression have provided me with a profound insight into living with them, which motivated me to search for further studies and research opportunities in order to contribute to increase the comprehension of these intricate and often misconceived conditions.

For instance, renowned psychologists such as Jordan Peterson and Aaron T. Beck indicated that there is a need to distinguish between the various types of attention deficit hyperactivity disorder, in order to comprehend better the impact of it on adults. Further, Marsha Linehan and Robert Sapolsky have both concluded that Cognitive Behavioural Therapy is advisable in order to alleviate symptoms of both anxiety and depression. It is similar to a jigsaw puzzle: with the interconnecting pieces, we are able to assemble a great deal of the picture, with what works best for managing these conditions.

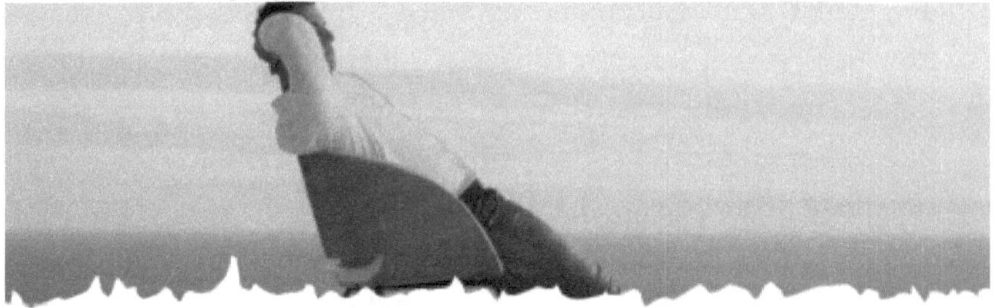

Through the often turbulent waters of mental illness, I have found ways to become more conscious of the effects of psychological disorders and manage the conditions more effectively. The various approaches I have taken have given me the opportunity to gain invaluable insight into the challenges that come with living with psychological disorders. This experience has inspired me to learn more by researching and studying psychiatry in greater detail and contribute to a growing understanding of mental health.

It Came Back

If it were not clear through this reading, my depression did indeed come back and I wanted to specifically speak to it as I don't want to fold it into the book where it is missed simply. Since the reality of it is, relapses are real, and although one could perceive me writing this book, I am far too aware and knowledgeable to have a relapse, but like you, I am human and I to fall down.

Life loves to pitch us curveballs when we least anticipate them. Despite the strides I had made in my recovery, a sudden shift occurred, and it felt as if depression had made a fierce comeback. I had been doing everything correctly, diligently adhering to my treatment plan and implementing lifestyle changes to bolster my mental health. Yet, depression managed to slip back into my life, casting a shadow on the progress I had worked so hard for.

My daily journal entries started reflecting changes in my mood and energy levels. Feelings of helplessness and frustration grew as depression seemed to regain control. Rather than giving in to these emotions, I chose a proactive approach to tackle this setback.

Through my research, I discovered that setbacks are par for the course in the recovery process. I learned that depression can be a recurring condition, and patience and persistence are key in managing it. This understanding motivated me to persist with my treatment plan and lifestyle adjustments while exploring additional strategies to aid my recovery.

I opened up to my psychologist about my struggles, who recommended incorporating mindfulness and meditation into my daily routine. This practice would increase my awareness of thoughts and emotions, allowing me to better handle the negativity associated with depression. My psychologist also suggested joining a support group to connect with others experiencing similar challenges and share our stories.

As I embarked on this new phase, I found comfort knowing I wasn't alone. Relying on my support system, including family, friends, and therapist, I continued to learn about depression and its many aspects. I stayed committed to daily journaling, which offered valuable insights into my thoughts and emotions while tracking my progress.

As days passed, my journal entries captured fluctuations in my mood and anxiety levels. Some days were better than others, but at times it felt like I was taking two steps back for every step forward. On high-anxiety days, even the smallest tasks seemed challenging. Walks with Winnie provided some relief, but not always enough.

My journal entries also documented the impact of external events on my mental health, like the passing of Eve's mom. The grief and stress of this loss compounded the challenges I was already facing. It was crucial on such days to recognize my limits and allow time and space for recovery.

Despite my frustrations with my progress's pace, I continued seeking support from mental health professionals. Conversations with Laree and Dr. P helped identify anxiety triggers and provided guidance on managing emotions. Dr. P advised adjusting my medication to prevent mania, illustrating that treatment plans can evolve to meet changing needs.

The funeral was particularly difficult, but medication offered temporary relief. However, the event's emotional toll left me feeling vulnerable, highlighted by a near-accident on the way home. This served as a stark reminder to prioritize self-care and be gentle with myself during trying times.

My journal entries depicted a person struggling to find balance amidst recovery's ups and downs. On some days, depression weighed heavily, tempting me to withdraw and abandon my goals. Yet, I continued to fight, finding solace in the support of loved ones and small daily victories.

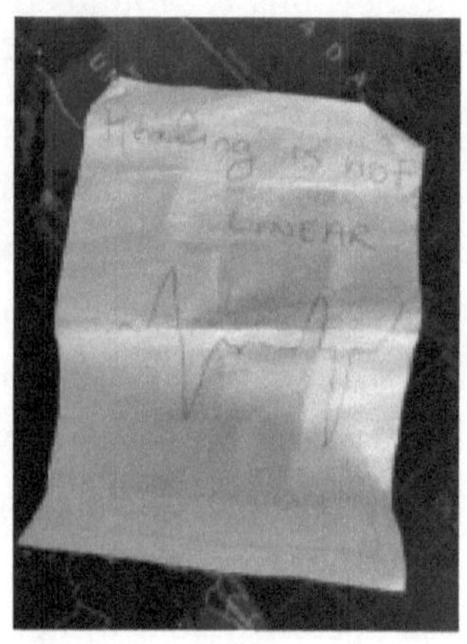

Recovery is seldom a linear journey, and setbacks are inevitable. I still have that piece of paper Dr. R gave me. By documenting my experiences and remaining committed to my treatment plan, I gained invaluable insights into my mental health and learned to adapt and persevere during the darkest moments. As I faced each new day, I clung to the hope that with time and persistence, I would eventually overcome my anxiety and depression, emerging stronger than ever.

Despite the unwelcome return of my depression, I refused to let it define me. I continued to take charge of my recovery, actively seeking new ways to improve my mental health and well-being. By sharing my experiences and being open to guidance, I demonstrated my determination to overcome this challenge.

In the end, it was this unwavering commitment to recovery that enabled me to face the return of my depression head-on, armed with the knowledge and tools to navigate the road ahead. And as I continued to make progress, I found hope and resilience in the knowledge that I could, and would, get better.

final thoughts

Despite managing difficult emotions, I feel appreciative of the education and understanding I have received as a result. I am truly excited to keep progressing, learning and developing more. This journey has demonstrated to me, and to those around me, that with the right attitude and reliable support, anyone who experiences the debilitating effects of anxiety, depression or ADHD can strive and achieve the goals they set out to reach.

As we come to the close of our discussion on the effects of severe depression, anxiety and attention deficit hyperactivity disorder, or ADHD, I must offer my gratitude to you, the reader, for joining me and giving this exploration so much meaningful attention. By piecing together the collaboration between our respective insights and real life experiences, we were able to gain a better understanding of the interactions between severe depression, anxiety, and ADHD. We figured out that understanding and dealing with these mental health issues requires resilience, self-awareness, and unwavering determination.

Whilst piecing this puzzle together, we also discovered that individuals living with mental health conditions have the strength and potential to live more fulfilling and brighter lives. This hope and internal healing can be achieved through psychoanalysis, coping mechanisms, and the assistance of close family and friends.

As we draw our time together to a conclusion, I wish to persuade you, the reader, to apply the lessons and understanding that we have established to the world around you. Let us continue to educate and spread awareness on the realities of those with ADHD, depression and anxiety. Create a communal atmosphere that implements understanding, kindness and compassion. Remind us all to be beacons of hope in a world that can, sometimes, appear dark.

Psychiatrists like Jordan Peterson, Aaron T. Beck, Marsha Linehan and Robert Sapolsky have all studied the effects of difficult mental health conditions and understand how deeply affecting it can be. For example, Robert Sapolsky, a neurobiologist from Stanford University, has devoted a lot of his life to studying how mental health and illness interact with everyday life. His work has shown us how most of the time we are able to look after ourselves, but on occasions in our lives when can't, it's important to ask for help. Drawing on personal experiences and research, Sapolsky has likened this journey to trying to find a way through a forest with a rope that has frayed halfway through, having to trim the rope every so often until you find your way out.

I thank you again, dear reader, for sharing in this exploration with me. This journey has been as beneficial to you as it has to me and continues to provide the strength and knowledge needed to create a brighter, more balanced future.

* 9 7 9 8 2 2 3 3 7 6 5 7 6 *